Reminiscence and
Life Story Work

of related interest

Remembering Yesterday, Caring Today
Reminiscence in Dementia Care: A Guide to Good Practice
Pam Schweitzer and Errollyn Bruce
Foreword by Faith Gibson
ISBN 978 1 84310 649 4

Reminiscence Theatre
Making Theatre from Memories
Pam Schweitzer
Foreword by Glenda Jackson MP
ISBN 978 1 84310 430 8

Reminiscence and Life Story Work

—— A Practice Guide ——

Fourth Edition

Faith Gibson

Jessica Kingsley *Publishers*
London and Philadelphia

First published in 2011
by Jessica Kingsley Publishers
116 Pentonville Road
London N1 9JB, UK
and
400 Market Street, Suite 400
Philadelphia, PA 19106, USA

www.jkp.com

Library of Congress Cataloging in Publication Data
Gibson, Faith.
Reminiscence and life story work : a practice guide / Faith Gibson. – 4th ed.
    p. cm.
Previously published under title: Reminiscence and recall.
Includes bibliographical references and index.
ISBN 978-1-84905-151-4 (alk. paper)
 1. Reminiscing in old age–Therapeutic use. 2. Older people–Psychology. 3. Social work
with older people. 4. Mentally ill older people. 5. Recollection (Psychology) I. Title.
BF724.85.R45G53 2011
362.6'6–dc22
                            2010050486

British Library Cataloguing in Publication Data
A CIP catalogue record for this book is available from the British Library

ISBN 978 1 84905 151 4

Printed and bound in Great Britain
by MPG Books Group

*To Mary Tara Marshall – valued friend
and creator of opportunities*

Acknowledgements

In preparing this fourth edition I continue to be indebted to many people, both directly and indirectly, for their help and encouragement. Special thanks to all who have shared their rich recollections with me over many years, either as individuals or as members of small groups.

I have taken account of other people's research, practice experience and writing, and have drawn on ideas from many sources. Exchanging ideas with other reminiscence practitioners and researchers has been immensely valuable but I take full responsibility for the views expressed and apologise if any acknowledgements have been inadvertently omitted.

Much of the material from the previous editions remains relevant. New insights, updated research findings, other authors' writing and continued teaching and practice experience with small reminiscence groups, life story work with individuals, structured life reviews and guided autobiographical writing underpin this new edition published by Jessica Kingsley Publishers, to whom I am much indebted for all their professional expertise and guidance.

I am grateful to Dorothy Atkinson, Michael Bender, Joanna Bornat, Mabel Cooper, John Killick and Pam Schweitzer for permission to quote from their own publications. The Marshall family has kindly given permission to quote from W.F. Marshall's poem.

The staff and members of the Northern Ireland Reminiscence Network are a source of continuing encouragement to me and I am especially indebted to Daphne Doran, Margaret Gordon and Rosemary and Nathan Hamill for much assistance and also my family and other friends who continue to reminisce and generously share their ideas with me.

Contents

——— *Chapter 1* ———

The Transforming Nature of Reminiscence

Reminiscence theory and reminiscence practice continue to develop. The power of reminiscence to transcend differences of age, culture, ethnicity, gender, geography, language, nationality, professional allegiance, politics and religion, once experienced first-hand, is an unforgettable experience. Reminiscence builds bridges between people. Through reminiscence – the sharing of memories of our personal life experience, with all their similarities and differences – we discover ourselves anew and encounter other people with enlarged understanding. We discover and rediscover the importance of relationships and recognise afresh our shared humanity with all its potential for good or ill. Far from locking us into the past, recalling and sharing memories brings new understanding, fresh perspectives, and courage for facing the future. The excitement of people new to reminiscence work as they discover these riches for themselves is a source of great satisfaction and pleasure for many people who have devoted much time and effort to developing and articulating the many varied aspects of reminiscence, life review and life story work undertaken with diverse groups and individuals.

Reminiscence and related narrative methods have achieved growing international recognition in recent years as research evidence of effectiveness slowly accumulates and the number of skilled practitioners grows. Its full potential to enrich, inform, and entertain, to transcend present limitations and to heal and improve present well-being and quality of life, however, are still under-utilised by too many people, especially older people, and those who live and work with them.

This is a book about creativity which brings growth and change for people of all ages. 'Creativity is the process of bringing something new into being' (May cited by Cohen 2000, p.12). It aims to encourage people of all ages to move beyond their present understanding of themselves by thinking again and consequently thinking differently about their past and therefore thinking differently about the present. It concerns various ways of recalling and thinking about the past so as to understand the present better. This book is informed by a developmental perspective which means that from early childhood through various stages into late life we have the capacity to grow, to change, to develop, and hence to move beyond where we presently are – not because we can change the past but because we can view it differently and respond to its influence in new ways. The more we understand the journey to the present, the more likely we are to be able to live with the present.

Reminiscence is both science and art and ongoing research is essential. Knowledge and understanding grow and develop each time people engaged in reminiscence critically reflect on that experience and share their ideas with others. It is this continuing development of knowledge, understanding and the ethical application of skilled practice which provides the justification for this new fourth edition aimed to update ideas about good practice. A developmental life span perspective provides the foundation for using reminiscence work, suitably adjusted, with people of all ages and varied living circumstances.

This book is designed as an introduction which will assist professionals drawn from numerous different backgrounds and also trained and supported volunteers to establish sensitive, responsive, reflective and reflexive reminiscence work for the mutual benefit of people of all ages, their families, friends, volunteers and professional staff. Reminiscence workers come from community arts, community development, health and social care, housing with care facilities, libraries, museums, schools, colleges, adult education and youth work. Oral historians may also find this a useful guide as it seeks to illuminate the many similarities and differences between reminiscence work and oral history in terms of objectives, values, persons engaged, scope and structure of encounters, types of records produced and the skills and techniques used.

The relevance of reminiscence in later life was emphasised in earlier editions more than in this edition, not because it has grown less relevant but because more is now known about the importance of memory and the relevance of reminiscence to so many other people of diverse ages. For this reason the contents have been substantially revised and expanded especially concerning life story work, and reminiscence related to people with depression, learning disability and those contending with palliative care and end of life issues. This edition reflects the growth of evidence-based research and more sophisticated understanding of the theoretical and practice implications of laboratory-based memory research, dementia and the residual resource afforded by procedural memory, the recognition of the significance of creativity in later life and the importance of cultivating memory in early childhood through engaging children in reminiscence conversation. Well established methods and techniques for using multi-sensory stimulation to achieve effective reminiscence and recall continue to be refined, while computer-assisted applications multiply. Reminiscence, a seemingly common or ordinary experience, continues to be an evolving dynamic area of psycho-social practice and related research is greatly enriched by the continued involvement of inter-disciplinary and multi-professional interests.

Using this handbook

Ideas about reminiscence and general principles concerned with how to do reminiscence work with groups, couples and individuals are explored in Chapters 2–7. Then Chapters 8–10 cover reminiscence and oral history in community development, with people from ethnic minorities, and intergenerational reminiscence. Chapters 11–15 deal with how to adapt the general principles of reminiscence work to meet the needs and circumstances of specific groups of people who have various disabilities like dementia, depression, hearing, sight and speech disabilities, learning disabilities or are contending with end of life issues and bereavement. Finally Chapter 16 considers staff development and training as well as issues concerned with quality, evaluation and research.

This chapter arrangement means that although a reader might wish to reminisce with an individual or a small group of people, for example older women who have dementia who attend a day centre, it is advisable first to read the earlier chapters before concentrating on the dementia chapter and so on. This sequence is important because the specific chapters build on the general knowledge and skills already covered in the earlier chapters. These general principles are not repeated again in the subsequent specialist chapters. Also, because every group consists of a collection of individuals, it is also helpful to read about working with an individual even if group work is intended. The ideas about stages or phases of work covered in Chapters 5 and 6 are equally relevant whether reminiscing with individuals, couples and small groups in domiciliary, day care, residential, family or community contexts.

There is much more to be learned about reminiscence work than can be covered in this introductory guide, but further reading – each chapter contains some suggestions – undertaking the application exercises and discussing reminiscence work with others will help reminiscence workers to make a start (Gibson 2004).

Conclusion

It is hoped that this handbook will help reminiscence workers to develop the attitudes, knowledge, understanding, values and skills needed to encourage people to value themselves by valuing their past. Whether undertaken by a paid carer, family carer or a good friend, reminiscence can enrich relationships, improve communication and enhance caring. This means that carers, as well as reminiscers, can benefit from reminiscence work.

Try to work through this book and its application exercises with a colleague or friend; discuss ideas with each other. It is also strongly recommended that an experienced reminiscence worker or other appropriate person should be used as a supervisor, consultant or mentor. Such a person can help develop understanding about the rewards and demands associated with reminiscence work and how it affects listeners as well as storytellers.

Training too is important as this aids the development of understanding about the needs, wishes and interests of the people involved in reminiscing as well as developing competence as a reminiscence worker. Apply ideas gained from reading as practice is essential in developing skills. By trying out the ideas, the first-hand infectious excitement of reminiscence will be experienced. Develop the habit of thinking back critically over each reminiscence session so as to become a better listener and more skilled in encouraging people to tell their stories. This is also a way of taking responsibility for personal learning.

Most people find it easier to do reminiscence work if it is shared with at least one other trusted person so that together workers share its ups and downs. They are then able to discuss what happens, constructively criticise and support each other, and through mutual help ensure that good quality reminiscence work becomes firmly established.

—— *Chapter 2* ——

Growing throughout the Life Cycle – A Challenge for All Ages

Learning outcomes

After studying this chapter you should be able to:

- understand how best to use this handbook
- appreciate the multiple, changing needs of people at different ages and stages throughout their lives
- realise the importance of recalling, reconstructing and sharing memories at every age
- become aware of why you want to encourage people to reminisce.

Learning to listen to people's stories

> Everyone has a story to tell,
>
> If only someone will ask
>
> If only someone will listen.
>
> (Anon)

This book is written for people who wish to value their own memories, learn about the advantages of encouraging others to remember their past lives, however long or short, and experience the benefit of sharing recollections with others. It is meant, especially for people who would like to know more about the importance of memory, the part played by reminiscence throughout life and how to use knowledge about a person's past to enrich life in the present. It is also relevant to everyone who would like to explore their own memories and record them in some tangible way so that they might be shared with other people now in the present and perhaps become a legacy for those who come after.

Regardless of age, almost everyone reminisces. Even very young children, adolescents and young adults reminisce. Although more concerned with reminiscing by older people, this book is not only about older people. It contains guidelines, suggestions rather than prescriptions or rules, to help develop good practice in reminiscence work with individuals, families, small groups and communities.

Whether a potential reminiscence worker or facilitator (these words are used interchangeably throughout) aspires to work with an individual or a small group in a person's own home, community club, day centre, care home, hospital, library or museum as a professional, relative, friend or volunteer, this book should help to develop high standards of reminiscence work.

It is important to remember two things about reminiscing. First, not everyone likes to look back and to recall the past, so a person's own wishes must be respected. If some people are not able to express their opinions clearly, either because of uncertainty about what is meant or because of communication problems, reminiscence must never be forced on them. People are usually able to show by their behaviour, if not in words, whether or not they want to reminisce. Second, if a person, of whatever age, is invited to talk about the past, there must have time to listen. Reminiscence is not a process to be rushed and everyone needs to be treated with great respect regardless of age and ability.

Views on ageing

A good place to begin is to examine ideas about growth, change and development throughout the life cycle by reflecting on different stages of development and the challenges which each stage brings. How people no matter what their age – child or adult – are treated will very much influence what they are prepared to share with others. Everyone of any age is a unique individual. In some ways, people might resemble others in their age group but in many more ways each person is different. The longer people live, the more likely they are to differ from each other. So never make the mistake of treating older people as if they were all the same. Everyone, whatever their age, has common human needs, but the way that these needs have been met or frustrated throughout life will largely determine what each person is like when they reach old age. Everyone is born with certain inherited characteristics and also with the potential to adapt to life's experiences. Then, depending on what happens to them, and how they respond, they reach late life with some degree of resilience, acceptance, contentment and a sense of coherence or well-being, or else they may feel demoralised, depressed, anxious, angry, critical, unhappy, disappointed and unfulfilled.

A person is very seldom all one thing or the other. Just as young children, adolescents and adults behave differently from time to time, so too most older people display a mixture of both positive and negative characteristics, depending on their genetic makeup (nature) and life's events (nurture). Health, education and economic and social circumstances, including satisfying relationships and living arrangements, past and present, all influence which characteristics and behaviour predominate at any time. In old age, a lifetime of experience with all its associated satisfactions and disappointments, together with present health and well-being, influence how a person seems at the present time.

Developmental psychologists emphasise the various stages everyone needs to work through, more or less successfully, or put another way the developmental tasks or challenges that are linked to each age stage of growth. Erikson (1982) suggests the eight stages listed below and the approximate age group to which they relate. This is a rough guide that identifies tasks or tensions and the stages identified tend to suggest a tidier, more orderly progression than actually occurs in real life. Taken overall, however, each stage or challenging tension needs to be satisfactorily addressed or resolved if a person is to successfully progress through the life cycle.

Trust – mistrust	Birth–18 months
Autonomy – shame	18 months–3 years
Initiative – guilt	3–5 years
Industry – inferiority	6–12 years
Identity – role confusion	12–18 years
Intimacy – solidarity	18–35 years
Generativity – self-absorption	35–65 years
Integrity – despair	65–death

Cohen (2000, 2005) expanded the brief reference Erikson made to the period from 65 to death by further developing ideas about the developmental and creative opportunities associated with the second half of life. Cohen proposed this period which spans some 40–50 years can be further divided into four, with each phase having distinctive challenges:

- Midlife re-evaluation – quest (40–60)
- Liberation – freedom (60–70)
- Summing up – meaning making
- Encore – life affirming legacy.

While much of this book refers to older people, it is essential not to see their needs in isolation from or as greater than those of other age groups but rather to appreciate the need to encourage solidarity, equality and friendship across all stages and ages of the life cycle. The interests of older people should always be situated within this broader framework which recognises the rights, needs and obligations of the whole human family which transcend both chronological and other boundaries. There are very practical as well as ethical reasons for suggesting this. Our society, along with most other developed and developing countries, is ageing largely because of falling fertility rates and because people are living longer. Solidarity between older people, their families and local communities is imperative. Only through such family, community, national and international solidarity are the health and social needs of the increasing number of very old people, including those who are physically or mentally frail, or both, likely to be adequately met.

Families have always been the major source of support both for older and younger people. This is unlikely to change in the foreseeable future despite many community care innovations and developments (Mandelstam 2010). Demographic changes, shifting public policy and increasing family mobility all combine to multiply the demands being made on neighbours, informal carers and volunteers. The survival of older people and the quality of their lives will increasingly depend upon their ability to find common cause with and assistance from those they live among. They need to be encouraged actively to pursue activities which help others to see them as constructive, contributing and valued citizens, eager to do what they can to assist others, rather than preoccupied with making demands on limited resources or boldly asserting their rights without also accepting obligations as fully participating citizens.

Promoting solidarity between the generations means that older people must be encouraged and assisted to remain socially engaged. They can best contribute to their own and others' well-being by involvement in a wide range of intergenerational activities, including undertaking adequately supported volunteering opportunities well matched to their interests and capacities, in addition to serving their own peer group, families and immediate neighbours.

Poverty, ill health and unequal opportunities throughout earlier life contribute to health problems in later life. Earlier adult life events such as unemployment, separation and divorce with their frequent consequences of poverty and social isolation, especially for women, chronic illness, including recurring mental illness, bereavement and prolonged caring responsibilities can all have deleterious long-term consequences. It is important in understanding people in the present to understand their earlier life experiences – their whole long journey to the present. The well-being of all citizens regardless of age is important and encouraging shared experiences across generational and other divides can have many wide-ranging benefits. Involving different age groups together by means of reminiscence activities can unite people across boundaries which otherwise tend to keep them apart.

Meeting the needs of older people

Age UK's *Age Agenda Bulletins* (2010) summarise the broad dimensions of current public policy, legal changes, reports and services concerning older people in the United Kingdom. It is important to provide good physical care for older people, including comfortable, secure, warm accommodation, acceptable food, and medical and social care, if required, but more is needed. A strong sense of personal worth and identity, with a conviction that essential aspects of life are still under one's own control, also influence how a person ages. In helping to provide love, security and a sense of belonging, carers and care environments can help people maintain their sense of worth, self-esteem, personal identity and well-being. In many ways, both large and small, older people and younger people too facing difficult challenges can be helped to feel in control of their lives rather than feeling marginalised or isolated. This is very important if they are to experience a sense of fulfilment, confidence, coherence and well-being throughout their lives.

Growing is a lifetime experience. People, whatever their age, can continue to grow and develop provided they experience the right nurturing conditions. For continued growth and development older people in particular need opportunities to experience:

- warm, caring relationships
- respect as unique individuals
- being listened to
- sharing and accepting their past life history
- being able to help others
- having genuine choices
- having spiritual and creative needs taken seriously
- interesting, stimulating activities so that they do not have to spend their days 'busy doing nothing'.

Reminiscence as explained in this book aims to help carers and others to become more competent in reaching out to people, particularly older people, in order to share their continuing journeys towards growth, development and personal fulfilment. It is especially concerned with recalling and re-working memories and how to encourage people to use reminiscence in making sense of their lives. It seeks to help workers discover and to value the interesting, intriguing, complex lives they and other people have lived; to use the past to enrich the present.

A lifetime of experience

There is much more to people than just what is visible in the present. No one, not even the apparently most 'ordinary' person, reaches late life without a tremendous variety of good and bad, constructive and destructive, positive and negative, rewarding and unrewarding experiences behind them. Everyone has lived an intricate, interwoven series of lives. For example, they will have played many parts as children, adolescents, students, friends, lovers, partners, parents, workers, grandparents, widows or widowers. To understand why someone is as they are now, perhaps in late life, it is necessary to know something about what has gone before and what meanings the person attaches to their life experience in the present. This means learning to listen to people's stories, to what is said, and also unsaid – to become finely tuned so as to be able to read the spaces or the silences between the words.

Reminiscence is a fruitful way of learning about such experience and its personal meaning. Through reminiscing, most people can be helped to review, re-work and re-evaluate their lives. This sharing process helps them to reconstruct memories, develop new perspectives, and become more accepting of life, however it has turned out – for good or ill.

Reminiscence may be very private but it is usually a two-way process in which people share recollections with each other. This mutual process then becomes a means of bridging the gap that so often exists between people of different ages, gender, social background, sexual orientation, class, race, politics, religion, education, status, position and power.

Often it is hard for younger people, whether they are professionals, family members or volunteers, to find things in common with people whose age and background differ markedly from their own. Middle-aged carers are frequently preoccupied with concerns about their own parents, their personal ageing or their own children. By becoming involved in reminiscence, experiences may be shared, relationships enriched and barriers overcome.

Use reminiscence to discover the rich, complex, colourful patterns of a person's whole long life. When this happens people are enriched and changed because they begin to share a journey which, while beginning in the past, takes place in the present; this becomes a journey which moves forward in new, exciting and unexpected directions.

Looking beyond the obvious

Age is not determined by years alone but depends, to some extent at least, on the interplay between how older people see themselves, how others see them, and the continuing opportunities they have to remain involved in life and engaged in loving relationships and satisfying activities or occupations. Health, income and satisfactory living arrangements all contribute to well-being. As Shakespeare said, in our time we all play many parts. We are likely to make more sense of the present – our own and other people's – if we have some awareness of what has gone before and how it has been experienced. The poem 'Kate' illustrates how important it is to look beyond present outward appearances and to appreciate the uniqueness of each person's life. It also shows how much Kate wanted her various pathways through life, her loves and losses, to be appreciated. She wanted her story to be known – but nobody had asked and nobody had listened.

'Kate – A Crabbit Old Woman'

What do you see nurse, what do you see?
What are you thinking when you're looking at me?
A crabbit old woman, not very wise,
Uncertain of habit with far away eyes,
Who dribbles her food and makes no reply,
When you say in a loud voice 'I do wish you'd try'.
Who seems not to notice the things that you do,
And forever is losing a stocking or shoe,
Who tries not to help you, try as you will,
With bathing and feeding, the long day to fill.
Is that what you're thinking, is that what you see,
Then open your eyes nurse. You're not looking at me.

I'll tell you who I am as I sit here so still,
As I rise at your bidding and eat at your will.
I'm a small child of ten with a father and mother,
And brothers and sisters, who love one another.
A young girl of sixteen with wings on her feet,
Dreaming that soon now, a true love she'll meet.
A bride soon at twenty, my heart gives a leap,
Remembering the vows that I promised to keep.
At twenty-five now I have young of my own,
Who need me to build a secure happy home.

A woman of thirty, my young growing fast,
Bound to each other with ties that should last.
At forty my young ones will soon all be gone,
But my man stays beside me to see I don't mourn.
At fifty, once more babies play round my knee,

Again we know children, my loved one and me.

Dark days are upon me, my husband is dead,

I look at the future, I shudder with dread,

For my young ones are busy, making homes of their own,

And I think of the years and the love I have known.

I'm an old woman now, nature is cruel,

It's her jest to make old age look like a fool.

The body, it crumbles, grace and vigour depart,

There now is a stone where I once had a heart.

But inside this old carcass, a young girl still dwells,

And now and again my battered heart swells.

I remember the joys, I remember the pain,

And I'm loving and living life over again.

I think of the years, all too few, gone too fast,

And accept the stark fact that nothing can last.

So open your eyes nurse, open and see,

Not a crabbit old woman, look closer, see me.

Conclusion

Reminiscence work with individuals, couples, families, small groups and communities is based on the conviction that people are best placed to know and to say what is important to them. Respectful, reflective listening can assist people at various stages of the life cycle to clarify and relate their own stories. The responsibility of the reminiscence worker is to enable them to engage in this process and to obtain satisfaction from so doing.

Key points

- To do effective reminiscence work it is essential to have a genuine interest in who people are and to enjoy reminiscing.
- Growth and development is a lifetime journey.
- Everyone fulfils many different roles and travels many different pathways throughout their lives to reach the present.
- People of all ages can enjoy reminiscing.

Application exercise

Whatever your age now, imagine yourself when old and consider how the answers to the following questions might contribute towards your having a sense of fulfilment and well-being. If you find this too difficult, think about a specific older person you know. Try to put yourself in the person's shoes (or chair). Then ask yourself these ten questions and write down the answers:

- Is he or she in good physical and mental health?

- Does he or she feel financially secure?

- Has he or she experienced a major change, illness, threat, move, trauma, poverty, discrimination, sexual abuse, loss or bereavement, particularly in the last few years?

- Does he or she have regular contact with a close friend, companion or confidant?

- Does he or she have regular opportunities for satisfying stimulation, occupation, interests and activities?

- How well are his or her care needs being met?

- Does he or she feel in control of his or her own life and present circumstances?

- What would be likely to give him or her great pleasure?

- What is the present state of his or her well-being?

- What are the major values that have underpinned his or her life?

Further reading

Age UK. *The Age Agenda Bulletins*. London: Age UK.

Coleman, P.G. and O'Hanlon, A. (2004) *Ageing and Development: Theories and Research*. London: Hodder and Arnold.

Gibson, F. (2004) *The Past in the Present: Using Reminiscence in Health and Social Care*. Baltimore: Health Professions Press.

Woods, R. and Clare, L. (eds) (2007) *Handbook of the Clinical Psychology of Ageing*. Chichester: John Wiley and Sons.

Chapter 3

What is
Reminiscence Work?

Learning outcomes

After studying this chapter you should be able to:

- understand four definitions of reminiscence
- appreciate how ideas about reminiscence have evolved over time
- justify the use of the term reminiscence work, not reminiscence therapy
- appreciate the wide relevance of reminiscence work.

Application exercise

- How would you describe or define reminiscence?

Before reading further, write down your own ideas. Then compare them with what others have said, as quoted in this chapter. Start with your own ideas first.

Four definitions of reminiscence

Different writers have defined reminiscence in various ways. Four widely used definitions are:

1. 'Reminiscence is the act or process of recalling the past.' (Butler 1963)

2. 'The recalling of memories from one's personal past.' (Webster 1997)

3. 'The process of thinking or telling about past experiences.' (Cappeliez, Lavallee and O'Rourke 2001)

4. 'Reminiscence therapy (with people with dementia) involves

the discussion of past activities, events and experiences with another person or group of people, usually with the aid of tangible prompts. The vocal or silent recall of events in a person's life, either alone, or with another person or group of people.' (Woods *et al.* 2005)

There are a number of important characteristics to note from these definitions:

- Reminiscence may refer to a single recalled memory or to a process or series of recalled memories.
- While reminiscence refers to the past, it occurs in the present and often looks to the future.
- The memories recalled relate to personal experiences or to the personal impact of public events.
- It may occur infrequently or habitually.
- It may be either a silent (internal) or spoken (shared social) process.
- It may be private or public – or a mixture of both.
- It may occur spontaneously or be triggered by some known or unknown stimulus.
- It may be opportunistic or purposely planned.
- It may involve little or considerable evaluation of the recalled memories.

Memories may remain private thoughts or be made public by being shared in various ways, mostly, but not only, as spoken or written recollections. While some recollections occur frequently, others only rarely come to mind. Some memories have very vivid specific details, sometimes called flash bulb memories but others remain hazy, vague and general. Memories are not static or fixed but are dynamic. That is why psychologists talk about memories, being constructed out of the interplay of stories, images in the mind and emotions which all come together to form personal autobiographical memories. The stories that we tell are formed out of our intentions at the time we are recalling the memories as well as from the original experiences. This means that each time a memory is recalled or rehearsed it will be changed to some extent (Rubin 1999). We reminisce to make ourselves more interesting to other people and more acceptable to ourselves. Constructing and sharing the stories both with ourselves and with other people helps us to accept with patience, humour and hope both other people and ourselves. One member of a reminiscence group said:

> Reminiscence makes you aware of who you are today and how you got there – I had not been willing to look at a part of my past life until I joined a reminiscence group and this made me realise I needed to face this thing, a personal thing, and I got on top of it. I never realised my memories were so important to me until I left home and started living on my own and had to manage everything for myself.

Reminiscence is a search for meaning – a search for understanding of our past. It is a re-tracing of where we have come from – a process for discovering and re-discovering who we are by making linkages between disparate aspects of our lives, our families and our communities. We come to understand as if for the first time, or to understand in different ways, the values, people and places which have shaped us and made us what we have become and are still becoming. For reminiscence is not the same as rummaging in the long neglected bottom drawer of a filing cabinet. It is not quite the same as leafing through the long ignored pages of a photograph album. It simultaneously invites reflection and reconstructing our memories. It is a means of becoming more contented with ourselves now and who we may become in the future.

A brief history of reminiscence theory and reminiscence work

The modern reminiscence movement draws from many different sources and disciplines for its inspiration, theoretical foundations and creativity. It draws ideas from different academic subjects including psychodynamic, clinical, cognitive and autobiographical psychology, anthropology, neurobiology and oral history. In developing ways of understanding and portraying people's memories it turns to the creative arts as vehicles for communication and representation including literature, drama, music, dance, photography and the graphic arts. As understanding of memory grows so too does skill in knowing how to stimulate and to use all the senses as pathways for accessing and recovering the rich deposits of personal memory. The significance of time, place, cherished artefacts and memorabilia of many kinds contribute to this seemingly ordinary, accessible and richly rewarding way of strengthening bonds between people.

Throughout history and in most cultures there have always been special storytellers as well as particular people who enjoyed passing on their experience to others by recalling the past. Some of these people wrote down their recollections while others relied on word of mouth. This oral transmission of traditions used to be called folklore or, more recently, oral history. For more information about oral history see Chapter 8. Although such activities were accepted by some, many professional clinicians believed that the tendency for people to reminisce more as they grew older, to 'live in the past', was a negative side of growing older. It was to be deplored, not valued, to be discouraged, not encouraged.

Slowly over the last 50 or so years the importance of being able to look back, to recall the past and to share recollections with other people has been recognised. Reminiscence, an everyday activity, used by most people of all ages throughout their lives, is increasingly valued and is now being widely used for educational, recreational, artistic, social and therapeutic purposes. Increasingly, writers emphasise the importance of understanding why many people of all ages, including children, love to talk about the past and why we benefit from telling our unique stories and having them heard by other people.

Kemp (1978), an architect, when working for the Department of Health in London, studied residential institutions for older people. He realised that, unlike many older people living at home, nobody in care homes and hospitals seemed to be talking about their past. Indeed many caring professionals at that time were actively discouraging such talk as they believed it interfered with an ageing person maintaining a proper grip on today's reality. Kemp's ideas challenged this belief. He persuaded Gordon Langley (Langley and Langley 1983), a psychiatrist, and a small team of artists and psychologists, to help him develop a reminiscence aid designed to encourage people in such facilities to reminisce. Help the Aged, who, in 1981, published the three-part tape/slide package *Recall*, carried Kemp's pioneering work forward. This audio-visual package dramatically stimulated the extensive development of reminiscence because busy staff in nursing and residential homes, hospitals and day centres now had a readily available and easily used working tool. Occupational therapists, psychiatric nurses and activity nurses, diversional therapists, among others, quickly recognised that reminiscence activities provided widely acceptable social and intellectual stimulation. Many other more local contemporary aids similar to *Recall* have been produced in the intervening years and many different paid and unpaid carers now use reminiscence in countless ways in their day-to-day work.

A number of American clinicians and researchers were already writing about the many different facets and functions of reminiscence some 20 years before this. Their work provided the early theoretical underpinning for the British and other work developing in other parts of the world including Australasia, Canada, Europe, Japan, South America and South Africa. The reminiscence training programme, theatre, exhibitions and publishing promoted by Age Exchange Reminiscence Centre in Blackheath, London, which was founded by Pam Schweitzer in the early 1980s, has had a major impact in developing reminiscence. Pam Schweitzer now coordinates the European Reminiscence Network that engages in trans-national action research and development projects; periodic intergenerational and international theatre performances; and publications, touring exhibitions and international conferences which provide a fruitful meeting place for academics, community artists, community development activists, health and social care professionals, oral historians, library and museum staff, older people, researchers, teachers, writers and volunteers.

Psychologists interested in autobiographical memory have sought to bridge the gap between laboratory-based cognitive experiments and understanding memory in real life situations. The International Institute of Reminiscence and Life Review provides a North American-Pacific Rim focus for the promotion and development of reminiscence research, publications and practice. Its biennial conferences are valued opportunities for researchers, clinicians and practitioners of varied backgrounds and nationalities to explore theoretical understandings and reminiscence practice across disciplines, including reminiscence, autobiographical memory, oral history and narrative methods which otherwise seem to inhabit largely separate and parallel worlds (Bluck 2009).

The increasing popularity of therapeutic reminiscence work has also coincided with a burgeoning interest in oral history, local history and family history. Historians are interested in making an accurate record of the past; they are less interested in the processes of remembering but have become increasingly aware of the effect on interviewer and informant of the interview experience and the ethics which should govern these encounters. They use focused oral evidence in seeking to understand and interpret history. For them, the outcome, most often an audiotape and transcript, is central. Because many reminiscence groups as well as interviews with individuals, although primarily concerned with providing personal fulfilment, communication and social stimulation, are also interested in producing a record of shared memories, the dividing line between reminiscence work and oral history is often blurred.

In oral history and folklore there are traditions of collecting and recording of memories, both with individuals and in groups, but the emphasis until recently has been more on recording individuals. Most reminiscence work is undertaken in small groups but individual work, often called 'life history', 'life story' or 'life review', is also increasing in popularity. As Bornat (2006), an oral historian and sociologist, suggested, reminiscence work, like oral history, can be thought of as a democratisation process – of giving people their place. In the health and social care services, reminiscence group work and also individual life story work is frequently used in many hospitals, care homes and day centres. Community arts organisations, community development agencies, voluntary community and social agencies, housing associations, museums, libraries, adult education groups, schools and colleges are actively pursuing reminiscence and allied activities either with mixed aged groups or with people of similar age who share common interests or face common problems.

With increasing numbers of frail older people continuing to live at home or with relatives, domiciliary carers and voluntary visitors also need to understand about the importance of reminiscence because they have many spontaneous opportunities to reminisce in their day-to-day contact and conversation with older people or while undertaking other care tasks. Sometimes they may also want to use planned reminiscence as part of a package of care to enrich communication, lessen isolation and provide constructive occupation. Family carers too can benefit by learning to use reminiscence but it is not always easy for them to find the time and energy required. More might be encouraged to do so if they were assisted by trained reminiscence volunteers. The increasing numbers of physically or cognitively frail older people living alone who are often socially isolated or lonely could also benefit from regular visits by volunteers trained to do life story work and some are beginning to have such opportunities.

Recognising the importance of the past has liberated both older people and their professional and family carers. People and professionals are now free to remember. As Dobrof, a social worker, said:

> In a profound sense, Butler's writings liberated both the old and the nurses, doctors and social workers; the old were free to remember, to regret, to look back reflectively at the past and try to understand it. And we were free to listen and to treat rememberers and remembrances with the respect they deserved. (1984, p.17)

Reminiscence is not limited to older people and those who have dementia. These are common misperceptions. Because of their increased free time and the life challenges they face, many older people do enjoy reminiscing and Butler (1963) suggested life review was a near universal experience of aged people. Depending upon their life circumstances and the associated developmental challenges presented, children and adolescents too as well as adults of all ages contending with varied transitions may also benefit from reviewing their past lives. By so doing they may resolve present problems and gain confidence to face future challenges.

Major characteristics of reminiscence

Reminiscence is usually cumulative with one memory leading onto another. One person's shared recollections frequently stimulate associated recollections in others, which in turn results in further details being remembered and more stories being recounted.

Both private and public reminiscence may be spontaneous and unintended, or memories and talk about memories may be purposely and deliberately encouraged and carefully planned. Whether recall is spontaneous or prompted may influence the memories recalled that may relate to either the distant or the recent past, to learned facts or to autobiographical life experience. This handbook is primarily concerned with encouraging good practice in prompted or planned recall about personal life experience but it also seeks to increase understanding about the importance of responding to spontaneously recalled memories.

By translating mental images into speech, writing, poetry, drawing, painting, drama, mime, music, dance or some other communication medium, the recollections have the potential to be shared with others and to give their owners additional benefits (Gibson 2004). This process of sharing enriches the experience for both teller and listener, providing the storyteller experiences the listener as genuinely interested, and totally without patronising condescension.

In the telling and retelling, the detail of a memory subtly alters. Both the context and the interaction between the teller and the listener influence the story. It does not matter if the details change with each telling. The process of recalling memories is more like painting a picture than taking a photograph as Pear (1922) suggested: 'the mind never photographs. It paints pictures' (Cited by Coleman 1986, p.2).Each time a picture is worked on, changes of light, mood and other circumstances will influence what is painted. Similarly, while the major characteristics or core of a memory remain recognisable, the fine details alter, reflecting differences of emphasis, mood, memory and interpretation. And memories are not neutral but come wrapped in emotion.

While most people enjoy reminiscing it is essential to remember that reminiscence does not suit everyone and it must never be hurried. Do not urge people to reminisce against their better judgement. Always respect their wishes. Also remember that people of all ages reminisce, not just old people. There is a widely held belief that older people reminisce more than younger people. This is probably not true for spontaneous recall by older people who are living active, independent, fulfilling lives. Recalling memories about the distant, rather than the recent, past possibly increases in older people whose present lives are bleak or boring, where nothing happens in the present worth recounting or where memories are being purposely prompted by the use of aids, props or triggers by reminiscence workers.

Not all reminiscence can be about happy memories because no person's life consists only of 'good old days'. Reminiscence recalls past pain as well as past pleasure, past loss as well as past joys. Reminiscence work is not about sentimental, nostalgic 'trips down memory lane' where the present is regretted and unfavourably compared with the past.

The modern reminiscence movement is primarily concerned with using recollection of past experience as a tool for coping in the present and anticipating the future. It is a dynamic, not a static, process which brings the past into the present and which constructs and reconstructs a newer version of memories recalled. Reminiscence workers need to be prepared for, and able to cope with, whatever kinds of recollections and associated emotions emerge. More guidance about coping with the recall of painful memories is given in Chapter 12.

Reminiscence therapy or reminiscence work?

This book does not talk about 'reminiscence therapy' although some writers, especially those employed in medical settings, do. Instead, the term 'reminiscence work' is preferred. This is because reminiscence is valued as a mutual process, a shared journey. People regardless of age who reminisce are not necessarily ill – although some may be – and awaiting treatment by expert reminiscence professionals, as the word 'therapy' implies. Rather, they are the teachers, witnesses, informants, authorities and custodians of invaluable information about their own past lives.

The task of a reminiscence worker is to encourage and assist people to share their life-long experience, their life stories, with themselves and with others, here and now, in the present. Although talking about the past, people are communicating in the present. In the process reminiscence workers will be enriched because they too become participants, not aloof, remote observers. Everyone involved, the storytellers, care staff, volunteers, family members, teachers and pupils, all can benefit from using this enjoyable everyday process. In many different ways, reminiscence is therapeutic, even though it is not strictly a therapy.

Reminiscence work employs many different approaches depending on the level of knowledge, skill, interests, confidence and experience of the people involved. It is not a neat set of precisely defined and rigorously tested techniques. There is no one universally agreed definition. Instead, it is a loose collection of ideas resulting in varied approaches, activities and practices that differ according to the specific objectives of the work, who is involved and where it takes place.

Reminiscence group work, individual life story or life history work and structured life review, all described in this handbook, differ from large recreational and social activities such as group excursions to museums, tea dances, fashion shows, mock weddings, old-time musical functions, sing-alongs and theatre and film shows, which usually involve much larger numbers of people. Within such activities, however, there will be many opportunities for spontaneous reminiscence, or these large events may be used as springboards for more intimate planned reminiscence work at a later time.

Different types of reminiscence work

In hospitals and care homes where people live in groups, and in day centres, reminiscence is usually undertaken as a small group activity. Some people, however, are much more suited to individual work and it is a mistake to assume that because people live in groups they should only be involved in group work.

It is helpful to distinguish between general or simple, and specific or special, reminiscence work.

General or simple reminiscence work

General or simple reminiscence work refers to well-planned work that uses mostly open-ended prompt questions or various multi-sensory triggers to stimulate recall on topics likely to interest all the participants and unlikely, as best as can be anticipated, to stimulate painful or long buried memories. Simple reminiscence usually employs readily available materials, or triggers, to encourage recall of accessible memories. This kind of reminiscence activity tends to aim at achieving sharing of common memories, sociability and educational and recreational objectives. It is more likely, but not always, to be undertaken in a group.

An example is a group of eight women in a care home who met with two staff members for ten weekly sessions to read aloud from library books, look at photographs and newspaper cuttings about women's work and to share memories about their own working and domestic lives.

Specific or special reminiscence work

Specific or special reminiscence work is more likely, but not invariably, to be undertaken with individuals or in small formed groups with closed membership. It requires careful selection of participants, clearly defined objectives and careful, focused, planned use of multi-sensory triggers or prompts designed to be of immediate relevance to the people concerned. It uses prompts known to coincide with the participants' past interests and is particularly, but not only, relevant to individuals who have dementia or are depressed, demoralised or unhappy. Such work is aimed at confirming personal identity, increasing self-acceptance, enhancing self-esteem, or possibly achieving behavioural change. It will involve deliberately encouraging personal life review and self-evaluation. Structured life reviews with an individual or guided autobiographical writing in a group are examples of specific work.

An example is a man with early dementia who attended a day centre. He was unhappy, aggressive towards other members and very isolated. A worker spent time twice weekly with him to encourage him to talk about his earlier family life, work and retirement. Together they wrote a life story book which contained photographs and certificates eagerly supplied by his family.

Depending on people's circumstances and needs, either simple or specific work may be more appropriate. Each approach requires skilled workers prepared to undertake careful planning, preparation, reflection on and evaluation of the work undertaken. Both approaches can considerably improve people's quality of life by enhancing communication and building relationships. Before starting, it is important for workers to decide what kind of reminiscence work is likely to be of most interest and use to the people and context in which it is being undertaken and what they feel able and confident to deliver.

Who should undertake reminiscence work?

This is an important question because some professionals may wish to claim reminiscence as their exclusive territory. Reminiscence is not the monopoly of any one profession. Many different people with assorted backgrounds employed in various types of organisations do reminiscence work. So, too, do volunteers or people with few recognised qualifications. Intergenerational work frequently involves teachers or youth workers. Family carers, friendly visitors and some domiciliary care workers are increasingly being encouraged to appreciate and to use the rich possibilities of reminiscence. Community artists, community development staff and adult educationalists are also increasingly attracted to reminiscence although they do not always describe it as such.

Attitudes, values, knowledge and skills are more important than any particular professional background. Reminiscence work is based on respect for each person's unique individuality; it recognises the interdependence of people within relationships and within families and communities. Skills can be learned, and those needed for effective reminiscence work include:

- active listening – 'listening with the third ear'
- empathising – sharing another's world without losing hold of your own
- attending – being available to people
- relating sensitively – not being a bull in a china shop
- being non-judgemental – accepting people as they are
- not being frightened by the expression of painful emotions
- being able to enjoy reminiscing and be interested in the past
- being disciplined, but willing to share personal stories
- being able to reflect upon, accept and offer criticism of the work done.

Conclusion

Reminiscence and life review mean different things to different people. This everyday common process is more complex than may first appear. Without a widely accepted standard definition it is not uncommon for people to use the terms reminiscence, life story work and life review in different ways, so before commencing such work it is important to be clear about what is being proposed and hoped-for outcomes. Each time people recount stories of their personal life experience the accounts will be influenced by variations in the recall process, present mood and circumstances and how the storyteller perceives the reaction of the listener. For this to be a satisfying experience the storyteller must feel respected and listened to and that the story being told is understood, believed or validated.

Key points

- Reminiscence and recall indicate mental health, not mental ill health.
- Some aspects and types of reminiscence resemble oral history.
- Reminiscence is more concerned with process than with achieving factually accurate history or tangible products.
- Not everyone wants to reminisce. Personal choice must always be respected.
- Reminiscence is undertaken with individuals, pairs or small groups.
- Memories have many facets, and may subtly alter in the telling.
- Some memories may be very painful to tell and painful to hear.
- Reminiscence is a process that must never be rushed.
- Reminiscence skills need to be learned through training, practice, reading, supervision, support and critical reflection.

Application exercise

Ask yourself the following two questions. Write down your answers. Try to find someone you trust and with whom you feel comfortable so that you can discuss your answers with them.

1. What aspects of reminiscence work appeal to me?

2. What aspects of reminiscence work worry me?

Further reading

Bornat, J. (ed.) (1994) *Reminiscence Reviewed: Evaluation, Achievements and Perspectives.* Buckingham: Open University.

Haight, B.K. and Webster, J.D. (eds) (1995) *The Art and Science of Reminiscence: Theory, Research, Methods and Applications.* Washington, DC: Taylor and Francis.

Webster, J.D. and Haight, B.K. (eds) (2002) *Critical Advances in Reminiscence Work: From Theory to Application.* New York: Springer-Verlag.

---- *Chapter 4* ----

Why Encourage Reminiscence Work?

Learning outcomes

After studying this chapter you should be able to:

- appreciate the challenges faced by older people in later life
- list reasons for doing reminiscence work with individuals, families, small groups and communities
- understand Webster's classification of the functions of reminiscence and Cappeliez's adaptation
- explain why it is important to set objectives for planned reminiscence work
- recognise different attitudes, styles and effects on morale of reminiscing.

Application exercise

Why do you think reminiscence work might be important? Begin by writing down as many reasons as you can. If possible, get a colleague to do the same and then discuss your reasons with each other.

Ten reasons for doing reminiscence work

There are many different reasons for doing reminiscence. These vary over time according to the needs of the people involved and the place or context in which the reminiscence takes place.

Reminiscence makes connections between a person's past, present and future

Our remembered past sheds light on the present and prepares us for facing an unknown future. It helps with problem solving. By looking back we are able to draw on evidence of past coping; we are encouraged in times present; and dare to hope we shall cope in the future. People of any age can be faced with a crisis which can threaten to overwhelm them. Events such as a serious illness or accident requiring admission to hospital, a relationship breakdown, divorce, bereavement, loss of home or job, leaving home or academic failure can all be experienced as major crises. For older people, increasing physical or mental frailty may result in them giving up their own home, moving into a care home or supported housing, attending a day centre, or facing up to other new experiences. Many will find their changed or diminished circumstances a daunting experience.

Remember how it feels to be 'new'. For example think back to starting school or starting a new job or going alone to some unfamiliar location or event. Put yourself in the shoes of someone who may have lost good health, independence, their own home, their lifetime partner, familiar places and possessions, and the comfortable routines of a lifetime. Reminiscence can help ease the anxiety of such major life events. It can assist people who are facing such challenges by encouraging them to draw on their past experience of coping and surviving.

Reminiscence helps people to think again and understand in a new way where they have come from and how they have got to where they now are, at whatever age and in whatever changing circumstances and challenging relationships.

Reminiscence encourages sociability and opens up new relationships

At a stage in people's lives when their social networks, meaning the significant people to whom each is connected, are probably shrinking because of death or changes in living arrangements, reminiscence may open up new relationships. It may help people to make new friends, or re-discover old friends, because it may help them see that other people have had similar experiences. They discover common ground or come to better understand the reasons for people being different. Talking about the past becomes an easy way of talking in the present, of discovering new resources in themselves and in each other.

Even if people live surrounded by others, in homes or hospitals, do not assume that this means they have close, supportive, warm relationships. Some will but others will feel isolated, lonely, sad and miserable. They may be grieving for lost places, lost people, lost things and lost independence. They may be struggling with coming to terms with how to lead private lives in public places. The challenge for care staff is how to help residents reconcile their need for personal privacy with their need for significant relationships. Both are important; both demand attention.

Joining a small reminiscence group may help solve this dilemma to some extent. In such a group people can share those parts of their lives that they choose to talk about. They remain in control of the story they tell, encouraged by the group facilitator or leader who enables them to talk each in their own way and in their own time. As they begin to trust the other group members they will feel more confident about moving from superficial conversation to talking about significant experiences. In sharing both pain and pleasure, hard times and good times, each person learns to accept themselves and others, and new relationships emerge.

This process of growing towards others through sharing deeply felt emotions is not limited to groups. It also applies to reminiscence work with individuals or pairs. The possibilities, however, are enlarged and multiplied through group experience. Here each member has the potential for becoming a resource to every other member while at the same time benefiting themselves. Groups offer the possibility of both giving and receiving.

As a care assistant in a care home said:

> We use reminiscence groups as a means of introducing a new resident and to help them feel at home with us. Reminiscence helps them find other people from the same neighbourhood with similar backgrounds to whom they can talk in familiar ways. It gets them over the strangeness.

Reminiscence confirms a sense of unique identity and encourages feelings of self-worth

A strong feeling of personal identity, of knowing who you are, gradually emerges in adolescence and young adulthood. This sense of identity is important at every age. It helps us to remain in control of our own lives and not be overcome by the pressures that allow us to be treated as if we were worthless human beings or just the same as everyone else. These issues may be more acutely felt in adolescence when young people struggle to establish themselves as independent self-directing persons and also re-emerge when advancing old age tends to threaten hard won independence.

Some people as they grow older feel they are no longer valued by others, and some find it difficult to value themselves. All too easily they accept the negative ideas or stereotypes that diminish their own significance and achievements, thus allowing themselves to be marginalised. Threats to self-esteem may be even greater for older people who during their lifetime have experienced ill-treatment, abuse, trauma, disturbed relationships, illness, immigration, racism and discrimination. By showing a genuine interest in the lives people have lived, by reminiscing with them, it is possible to rekindle or reinforce a sense of uniqueness, of personal identity and self-worth. People will come to value themselves in the present and by feeling more in control of their own lives their present well-being may be safeguarded.

Reminiscence assists the process of life review

The term 'life review' is used loosely as a general term and also in a more technical way (see Chapter 7). In general, many people as they grow older become increasingly aware of past experiences, especially painful, difficult, unfinished business or unresolved conflicts. As Erikson (1982) suggests, everyone has particular tasks to work on at different stages in their lives. The task or challenge that faces older people is to negotiate the tension between integrity and despair, to come to terms with life as it has turned out – for good or ill. Some become increasingly aware of trying to review, resolve, reorganise, reintegrate and tidy up their past experience in the face of encroaching age and approaching death. Dealing with the past becomes a part of preparing for death (see Chapter 15).

It does seem that for many, but not all, older people, if they can be helped to take a second look at their past, to 'put their house in order', they develop a kindlier view of themselves. They can be helped in this process of life review by affirming that their life has been significant. In becoming easier on themselves, many become easier on others around them. Dealing with the past makes life in the present more understandable, more bearable.

Reminiscence challenges the distribution of power

Reminiscence can be a most effective tool for improving communication and increasing empathic understanding. By telling their stories, people reach out to others while reaching deep within themselves. A life story creates, sustains and alters relationships.

In almost all residential institutions (and in families too) there is a pecking order. Everybody, staff member, family member and resident alike, has their 'place'. Staff are always more powerful than residents. People with dementia are especially likely to experience a loss of significance or importance within their own families, in health and care establishments and in the community. Reminiscence work, however, in which residents, family members, volunteers and paid carers share experiences, will help restore a sense of personal significance. In this sense reminiscence work empowers older people and others who feel ignored or demeaned.

In understanding a person's past, it is easier to understand their present behaviour – even troubling and troubled behaviour. People become more finely tuned to each other's needs, more accepting of them and more able to reach out to each other. By reminiscing together, people learn to trust each other more and become less preoccupied with position, power and protocol. In this sense, reminiscence can have far-reaching, radical implications and consequently not everyone welcomes it. In the words of a young care assistant:

> Since I started working with Brian on his life story book I feel we have begun to respect each other – we are sort of more equal. He no longer seems to need to put me down the way he used to when he always called me 'that wee girl' and this made me try to boss him around. We are now much more relaxed with each other, and I no longer feel I have to prove myself to him.

Reminiscence encourages communication and assists staff development

When first meeting someone, regardless of age, it is nearly impossible to understand why the person is as they now appear. Everyone travels many journeys to reach the present and some of these journeys are harder than others. Past experience leaves its mark. By listening to people reminisce, these different journeys emerge and so it becomes easier to understand the traveller in the present. Because the person is seen differently, he or she will be treated differently. When each person is treated as a unique individual, understanding is increased and sympathies are enlarged. Reminiscence workers can help celebrate and value the heroism of lives remembered. If, on the other hand, the reminiscence reveals suffering caused to others in the past, the worker will need to distinguish between accepting the person and not accepting the past behaviour. It will be important to listen to the story, if possible helping the teller to find forgiveness, make restitution, and resolve or integrate the hurt or pain remembered. One manager of a care home said:

> I never understood why Hugh was so difficult, why he hated being here so much, until I heard him talk about his childhood. Now I see him differently, I understand him more and we have something to talk to each other about.

If in the course of reminiscence or life story work a facilitator becomes aware of information that may have criminal or legal implications, guidance should be sought from line managers, trade unions or professional bodies. Reminiscence workers, either paid or unpaid, must abide by the policies and practices of their employing or sponsoring organisations and the ethical codes or guidelines of relevant professional associations (Northern Health and Social Care Trust 2009).

Reminiscence aids assessment of present functioning and informs care plans

If health and social care staff only consider how a person presents in the present, it is like taking a single snapshot instead of looking through a whole photograph album. It is not a fair way to assess a person's present capacities. It is impossible to understand them now without knowing what they used to be like, what they used to be able to do, and liked to do, what values influenced them, and what they desired for themselves and their families. Their history suggests what they may still be able to do and what might still interest them, given half a chance. Reminiscence helps fill out the details of a person's life history in a fuller way than a clinical history which aims to gather information relevant to specific conditions or illnesses. A life story based on reminiscence helps illuminate why a person is as they are in the present. It is vital that assessments and care plans are based on all relevant information, relating to both past and present, because judgements made by professionals can have profound consequences for influencing ill-being or well-being of people receiving health, housing and social care services.

In some care homes, reminiscence with a key worker may be an established way of contributing to assessment, developing a care plan and helping newcomers settle. Life stories reveal how people think about their own lives and what meanings they attach to life. The process of gathering a life story helps the carer to grasp the essence of the other person and to understand how that person views the present changed circumstances in the light of lifetime values and experience.

Reminiscence reverses the gift relationship through teaching, preserving and transmitting knowledge and values

Those who have lived history are its best teachers. Bearing witness is important to many people as they grow older, and reminiscence may be described as seeing and seeing again, of telling and telling again.

Older people are irreplaceable sources of historical knowledge and, given encouragement, many are prepared to share their experience and wisdom with younger people. Instead of being passive recipients of others' caring, of having things done for them and to them, through reminiscence they are able to move to the centre of the stage. As soon as older people become the teachers, their families and carers become the learners. In letting an older person become the authority, the hearer becomes the student. The teller becomes the giver while the listener becomes the receiver or beneficiary. So reminiscence connects older storytellers to their earlier lives, to their contemporaries and to younger generations.

Each time an old person dies, history dies with them. A book is lost. This loss is felt most acutely by close family members. Families who discover and preserve their family history before it is too late are immensely enriched; they gain an invaluable legacy but also great mutual satisfaction and shared pleasure between the generations. One bereaved family carer said:

> Why did I leave it so late? I always meant to get Mum to tell me about the family but I never got around to asking her. When I was younger I was bored by her stories. When I was older I was too busy to bother. Now she's gone and we've lost her and we've lost the family history too.

Many people find they are ambivalent, if not apprehensive, about making the transition from employment to retirement. Frequently the advantage of having increased leisure, even at the expense of reduced income, causes apprehension rather than pleasure. Encouragement to explore personal and family history at this time can be both absorbing and helpful. Researching, writing or recording memories in one form or another releases energy and opens up new interests. Discovering long lost or little known aspects of family connections can be very exciting. There are many possible sources of information including census, cemetery and church records, ships' passenger logs, veterans' records, birth, death and marriage records and many relevant websites. Such genealogical research is likely to trigger personal reminiscence as well as providing fresh avenues for social and intellectual exploration, personal awareness and often new or renewed family connections. It can also be closely linked to autobiographical writing and structured life review resulting in greater personal awareness and acceptance of one's life (see Chapter 7).

If we learn to listen to people remembering and remember ourselves, we capture the past. If we tell someone else and record or write down the recollections, we help to preserve the past and transmit the culture. This applies as much to domestic history as to national history. One is the record of so-called ordinary people telling about their ordinary lives. The other concerns national or public events which people witnessed at first hand, or the times they lived through when such events occurred. Bornat (2006) writes about reminiscence as a social movement because reminiscence gives a voice to those not usually thought of as opinion formers. It provides raw material for oral history that Thompson (2005) persuasively argues has now become a respected part of historical studies.

Reminiscence contributes to social inclusion and community development

Many neighbourhoods and communities lack a sense of social cohesion and shared values with different groups within them experiencing isolation, marginalisation and discrimination. Reminiscence and oral history groups can provide a focal point for isolated or disaffected people. Groups who do not usually mix can be encouraged by means of local history projects or adult education classes in which reminiscence plays a part, to discover common experiences and mutual interests, thereby lessening suspicion and fostering shared understandings.

As well as stressing the importance of recognising the unique individuality of each person, it is also essential to promote better relationships within communities and between groups who may differ in age, ethnicity, religion, culture, language and politics. Exchanging personal and communal histories is one way of discovering what hopes and aspirations people share, of encouraging friendships and building cohesive, responsive services. People do not have to remain captives to history and heritage; difference can be respected and celebrated and become a force for good rather than division. The history and repetitive character of much community conflict and suspicion can be discussed and re-evaluated. Reminiscence undertaken within a community development framework is more often described as oral history but its objectives and many of the methods used closely resemble reminiscence work.

Reminiscence and related activities are relatively easy to undertake, economical, low risk and are widely enjoyed

This does not mean that all reminiscence is happy. Some recollections will be happy, others sad, although such recollections can be very helpful for some but not for all people. Not everyone wants to reminisce. It is crucial that any reticence or reluctance is respected. Some people can only keep the painful past in its place by ignoring it. Others may be so taken up with living in the present and thinking about the future that they have no time or desire to think about the past.

Different attitudes and reactions to reminiscence

Research by Coleman (1986), a psychologist, showed that different people use reminiscence in various ways. Table 4.1, based on his findings, is a reminder that reminiscence does not suit everyone.

Table 4.1: Morale and types of reminiscers		
1. Reminiscers	People who value memories of the past	High morale
2. Reminiscers	People troubled by memories of the past	Low morale
3. Non-reminiscers	People who see no point in reminiscing	High morale
4. Non-reminiscers	People who avoid reminiscing because of the contrast between their past and present	Low morale

Source: Adapted from Coleman (1986, p.36).

So it is very important to understand people's perspectives on their life stories and the different outcomes from sharing them. For the first group of people identified in Table 4.1 who reminisce readily, their memories are a source of strength which they and reminiscence workers can use as a resource in the face of present difficulties. If faced with problems, a reminder that these people have coped in the past may help encourage them to draw on evidence of past coping to overcome present problems. Being reminded of the past is likely to help them to value and use this experience in the present.

The second group brood on their memories, feeling regretful and sad. Try to gauge how rational or irrational such regrets are. Counselling may help these people to view their past and their perception of it somewhat differently. Some people will have very good reasons for feeling guilty about their past. They may feel even worse if the person they have wronged or ill-treated is now dead, so it may not be possible to make amends. These troubled people may like to talk with a minister of religion or a counsellor, who may be able to help them to move from a sense of guilt to a sense of forgiveness and acceptance.

The third group should be helped to get on with the things they consider are important to them. They should not be forced to contemplate their past. If they are 'doers', the challenge is to let them find satisfaction in whatever is important to them, here and now.

The fourth group say their past lives were happy, but reminiscence makes them sad when they do not necessarily need to be, so they avoid thinking and talking about the past. Unless these people can come to terms with the changes and losses in their lives, they are likely to remain depressed or unhappy.

Webster's classification of reminiscence functions

Webster (1997, p.140), a psychologist, has developed a Reminiscence Functions Scale (RFS) from which he derived eight separate factors representing the main functions of reminiscence:

1. boredom reduction – having something to do
2. death preparation – valuing the life lived and becoming less fearful of death

3. identity preservation – discovering and better understanding a sense of who we are

4. problem solving – drawing on strengths and experience from the past for coping in the present

5. conversation – rediscovering common bonds between old and new friends

6. intimacy maintenance – remembering personally significant people who are no longer present

7. bitterness revival – sustaining memories of old hurts and justifying negative thoughts and emotions

8. teaching/informing – teaching younger people, including family members, about values and history.

Cappeliez, Guindon and Robitaille (2008) and Cappeliez (2009) re-grouped Webster's eight functions under three headings as follows:

1. Private reminiscence with positive outcomes
    • Identity preservation
    • Problem solving
    • Death preparation

2. Private reminiscence with negative outcomes primarily serving the person
    • Boredom reduction
    • Intimacy maintenance
    • Bitterness revival

3. Public interactive pro-social reminiscence with positive social outcomes
    • Conversation
    • Teaching/informing.

For many people and their carers reminiscence, especially in groups, gives intense pleasure, excitement and enlightenment. For others it is a diversion, a means of reducing boredom, of passing the time. For most it is a constructive occupation which can readily lead on to many other related creative activities (Craig 2005).

Different styles of reminiscing

Fry (1995) suggested that people have different styles of reminiscing. As they tell their life story, the careful listener comes to understand whether the teller uses reminiscence in an affirming and positive way or in a negative, despairing way.

People with an affirming style accept both positive and negative life experiences. They are able to face conflicts or problems and to feel reasonably hopeful that the difficulties can be resolved. They have a sense of wholeness or coherence about their lives.

People with a negative style of reminiscing present life as gentle and pleasant. They ignore or play down or wall off painful or traumatic experience, and often recall public rather than personal experience as a means of distancing themselves from the impact of talking about their intimate past; they play it safe.

A despairing style means that the person is painfully aware of, and probably preoccupied with, conflicts and past and present negative experiences. These feelings emerge as a lack of fulfilment, pain and disappointment that the person seems unable to repress, deny or grow beyond.

Conclusion

Although reminiscence is a very common everyday experience, engaged in by most people from time to time, it is not as simple as it first seems and it is not universally helpful to encourage it. The immense importance of being able to remember, however, is summed up by McConkey (1997) who suggests that personal identity is dependent on memory because memory makes it possible to connect the past with the present and assists in making sense of our lives.

Key points

- The functions served by reminiscence will differ from person to person and for each person over time.
- Various researchers have formulated these functions in different ways.
- Not all the functions identified apply to everyone or to the same person all the time.
- Try to understand what reminiscence means to you and to each individual at the life stage each has reached and in the present circumstances.

- Identify different styles of reminiscing in other people and think about your own reminiscing style.

- Develop curiosity about your own and other people's past lives. Do not see yourself and them only through 'present spectacles'. Try to locate them and yourself within an overall life span that stretches from birth to the present and projects into the future.

- Be sensitive to people who need to forget rather than to remember. Respect their wish to live in the present and not to talk about the past.

Application exercise

1. Now that you have read this chapter, think of three people of any age you know who enjoy reminiscing. Write down why you think reminiscence is important to each person and why reminiscence is important to you.

2. Could you draw a timeline for yourself, marking in the major events so far in your life? Think about why you have chosen these events as being of major importance (see Chapter 7).

3. Do you know enough about the life history of the three people you identified to enable you to draw a timeline of their lives?

4. Discuss your work with a trusted colleague.

Further reading

Bender, M., Baukham, P. and Norris, A. (1998) *The Therapeutic Purposes of Reminiscence*. London: Sage.

Cappeliez, P., Guindon, M. and Robitaille, A. (2008) 'Functions of reminiscence and emotional regulation among older adults.' *Journal of Aging Studies 22*, 266–272.

Hendricks, J. (ed.) (1995) *The Meaning of Reminiscence and Life Review*. New York: Baywood Publishing.

Webster, J.D. and McCall, M.E. (1999) 'Reminiscence functions across adulthood: A replication and extension.' *Journal of Adult Development 6*, 73–85.

--------- *Chapter 5* ---------

How to Begin Reminiscence Work – The Planning Phase

Learning outcomes

After studying this chapter you should be able to:

- understand about phases or stages of reminiscence work with individuals, couples and small groups
- identify the responsibilities of senior staff in facilities where reminiscence and life story work is to be undertaken
- be aware of the overall responsibilities of reminiscence workers
- appreciate the importance of the preparation or planning phase in reminiscence work
- summarise the reminiscence worker's tasks related to the planning phase.

Phases or stages of reminiscence work with individuals, couples and small groups

Reminiscence work is the term most commonly used in reference to reminiscing in small groups and life story work more often refers to reminiscing with an individual. Life review usually refers to the evaluative element within either group or individual work or to specific types of reminiscence intervention (see Chapter 7). Aspiring reminiscence workers who are unaccustomed to doing group work will find it helpful to read a general group work text as here it is only possible to provide a limited introduction (Benson 2010). All planned reminiscence work whether it is undertaken with an individual, a couple, a family, a small group or as a larger community project moves through different phases or stages, overall from beginning

50

to end. This idea of structure although borrowed from group work writing applies to all planned time-limited reminiscence and life story work, regardless of the number of people involved. Writers use different words to describe these rather untidy and often overlapping stages. All agree that it is important to understand what happens in groups or a series of planned sessions with an individual or couple throughout the lifetime of the reminiscence engagement because workers and participants behave differently at each stage. Roles, tasks, responsibilities and relationships also change at different stages.

The amount of time or number of sessions within each stage varies according to the total time involved throughout. Within each single session, group meeting or a project's lifetime similar stages apply so it is a useful way of structuring encounters and of identifying tasks, responsibilities, behaviours and emotions of members and leaders which change during the different stages of the reminiscence work. Tuckman and Jensen (1984) suggested all groups pass through the following five stages:

1. forming
2. storming
3. norming
4. performing
5. adjourning.

'Forming' is the stage of getting together, beginning to get acquainted, making trial and error suggestions, and much indecision. 'Storming' is the stage when rules and boundaries are tested, anger is often expressed and conflict recognised. The group then emerges into the 'norming' stage where agreement is reached about how members will work together, plans are formulated, and trust starts to grow. This is followed by the 'performing' stage that sees tasks accomplished and satisfying relationships or group coherence established. Long after his original formulation Tuckman added a final stage of 'adjourning' when tasks are completed and the group disbands.

Shulman (2006) identified four stages or phases:

1. preliminary–preparation and planning
2. beginnings
3. middles
4. endings

Few groups behave in as neat and orderly a way as these two lists suggest. Most groups are more likely to progress in a cyclical rather than a linear fashion but it is still helpful to think about stages and this handbook uses the Shulman terms as they particularly allow the responsibilities of group facilitators to be described in detail and can also be used to guide reminiscence work with individuals or pairs. The success of any reminiscence work largely depends on how carefully the leaders or facilitators plan and prepare for it. Careful preparation overall and for each session is important with the early and late sessions requiring special attention. The beginnings and endings of a project and also of each separate session are times of heightened emotions and expectations and consequently they provide important opportunities for work which requires the facilitator to be finely tuned to the feelings of the participants.

Models of group work

Just as people have different styles of reminiscing, so groups differ depending on their objectives, leaders' ideas about group work and members' characteristics. There are many different kinds of groups, models of group work and styles of leadership. Distinctions between models are not always as clear cut as some writers suggest. One appropriate model for reminiscence group work is described as a 'mutual aid' group. This means a group where members are encouraged to join in shared discussion as equals on freely agreed topics and to behave according to mutually acceptable guidelines or ground rules. The leader acts as an enabler or facilitator, not an authority. The leader or worker is responsible for creating a safe place within explicitly agreed boundaries and for encouraging members to share their life experience with each other. The discussion focused on recounting experiences and feelings or emotions associated with those recalled memories within a warm supportive group is known as the group process. This is the most important aspect of what happens in a reminiscence group. In this kind of encounter, reminiscence is used as a vehicle for achieving communication and providing mutual support as well as various benefits for each individual person.

Some reminiscence work whether with individuals, couples or small groups is better described as an 'activity' or as 'task centred'. Here the emphasis is on 'doing', on producing a tangible, visible outcome. The reminiscence activity is important in itself but in this type of group it is a means to an end. This approach concentrates on achieving an agreed outcome or a specific product.

Most local and oral history work devoted to recording, writing and publishing people's memories fits this category. Objectives may be quite specific such as preserving history by means of sound or video recording, writing a family history, or publishing a record of a local neighbourhood during an identified period. Some people may wish to become historical informants and pass on their knowledge and experience to families, students and researchers. Some groups will want to achieve a single event such as an exhibition, a reading of their written work or a play or performance based on members' recollections to which others are invited. Some may wish to establish a database or an archive. Reminiscence becomes part of the means for achieving these possible outcomes. A list of such possible products produced by groups or individuals is given in Chapter 7, Table 7.1.

Reminiscence work with an individual, couple or group may have a single major emphasis, but seldom are other aspects totally excluded. Many reminiscence groups in care settings, for example, begin as mutual aid or 'talk' groups with process or discussion being emphasised but, during their lifetime, members may decide to write down, record, publish, illustrate, perform or exhibit the outcomes of their discussions. In such groups both the process and the product are important. In other groups which initially set out to be task centred, members usually gain additional intangible benefits such as warmth, acceptance, friendship, social confidence and improved self-esteem, as their life experience comes to be heard and appreciated by others, and incorporated into a tangible product which can continue to reinforce these positive outcomes.

Reminiscence, once begun, develops a dynamic of its own. If a show, book, exhibition or other product is produced, it in turn will stimulate further reminiscence by the audience, reader or viewer. So the process once begun will have many different and frequently unforeseen outcomes for people far beyond the group responsible for the initial production.

Reminiscence therapy

Some reminiscence work undertaken by professionally qualified therapists or counsellors, in which recall and review of the past play a large part, is described as 'therapy' or 'psychotherapy'. Groups led by trained psychotherapists are called psychotherapeutic groups. This approach aims to help members uncover complex, painful, perhaps long-buried memories and unresolved conflicts that 'leak' into the present and interfere with present functioning, adjustment and well-being. This book does not attempt to equip people for such highly skilled work which requires clinical professional training and close supervision. Whatever the objectives and emphasis within reminiscence work, if it is a positive, nurturing, constructive experience, freely entered into, for participants it will indeed be 'therapeutic' although not labelled a 'therapy'.

Responsibilities of senior staff

Managers in care homes, hospitals, supported housing facilities, day centres, libraries, museums and community arts organisations are in key positions to encourage and support reminiscence work. They have the responsibility to ensure that the needs of people served by their organisations for acceptance, warmth, respect, social and intellectual stimulation, companionship and fulfilling activities are sensitively met. They are responsible for creating a climate in which people feel valued and their life experience validated. If they set the lead, other staff will follow. Reminiscence work will happen, and be done well, or will not happen, or be done badly, depending on the lead given by managers, the commitment they make and the resources they command.

Managers should identify other staff members who share their concerns, so that together an active participative environment where each person is recognised as a unique individual with a long and interesting life history is created. Reminiscence work will flourish only if senior managers affirm its importance, staff are allowed time in which to do it (including time for preparation, de-briefing and supervision) and feel they and the work they do is valued.

In reminiscence work continuity of leadership that allows trust within a group or with an individual to develop is important. Managers must make sure that if staff are committed to an agreed number of reminiscence sessions or interviews, then duty rotas and workload management will enable them to be available at the agreed times. If the arrangements for reminiscence sessions are casually altered, participants will feel the work undertaken and the memories recounted are also regarded as of little consequence. As far as possible, managers must also ensure that participants as well as staff are free from competing or conflicting demands which may make it hard for them to attend at regular times.

Some staff, regardless of responsibilities and seniority, may not be convinced about the importance of reminiscence work. As McKee *et al.* (2003) reported, 'just chatting' is not highly valued, especially in residential and nursing facilities, although residents regard it as enormously important. Staff may be sceptical about the value of taking time to reminisce and critical of colleagues for wanting to spend time on something they regard as a 'soft option' or not 'real work'. This important point about sabotage is further developed in Chapter 11 in relation to people with dementia. Staff will quickly take their lead from managers. If they see that senior staff value reminiscence and enable it to happen, they will be less likely to contribute to its disruption.

All staff members need to understand the importance of reminiscing and be equipped to respond to spontaneous reminiscence in sensitive ways. Those who wish to develop reminiscence skills should be encouraged to do so by being trained and involved in more formal planned reminiscence work. Everyone in a facility, however, can contribute in one way or another. All can be involved, for example, in responding to spontaneous reminiscence, assisting in locating materials, lending objects, making suggestions, and sharing in celebrating outcomes.

Consciousness-raising sessions about reminiscence work for all staff – administrative, care, domestic, management and maintenance – are recommended (Gibson 2004). This is one way of identifying interested individuals who could then be offered basic training and so progress to facilitating reminiscence work. If a manager is introducing reminiscence work for the first time, it is helpful to discuss the idea at a staff meeting. Some knowledge about the importance of valuing people's memories and how planned reminiscence and life story work are usually undertaken is important for all staff. The implications for participants, their families and staff should also be discussed and ideas shared about how everyone might contribute.

If high standards of reminiscence work are to be achieved, supervision of workers is essential. Managers either need to take responsibility for this supervision and oversight or else ensure that alternative arrangements are in place. Chapter 16 contains more information about various ways of providing supervision and support and the potential of reminiscence work as a staff development tool.

Choice of facilitators and possible participants, practical details and issues of confidentiality will all require detailed discussion in the staff group. Agreement about what information arising from the reminiscence work will be shared, with whom and in what format is also important.

Some of the major questions to be agreed about sharing information include:

- Who will have access to it?
- Will it be included in care plans?
- Who will be responsible for writing the care plans?
- Who will be entitled to read such plans?
- How will participants be involved in consenting to this record keeping process?
- What less formal and more accessible way might also be developed, with consent, to acquaint staff with brief summaries of relevant information arising from reminiscence to better inform their care?

The responsibilities of reminiscence workers or facilitators

Many different reasons for encouraging reminiscence have already been summarised. Reminiscence practitioners need to think carefully about the people they hope to work with. They may decide to concentrate on only some of the objectives listed as it will be unrealistic to aspire to fulfil all the aspects mentioned in Chapter 4. Depending on experience and interest, reading the chapters about reminiscence with people with disabilities is recommended before deciding who to reminisce with and for what purposes. The general principles outlined in this chapter will need to be modified when working with people with particular impairments. Reminiscence practitioners need to be selective about what they hope to achieve in any particular reminiscence project or group, remembering that needs and interests of both individual members and the group as a whole may alter over time.

Preparation or planning phase of work

Meticulous planning and preparation will largely determine whether or not the work attempted is effective. Planning nearly always takes much longer than novice workers anticipate. Before starting any reminiscence project or group consider the questions listed below. It is not sensible to give stock answers to these questions but general guidelines will encourage workers to find their own answers. Preparations will depend upon the desired objectives, the characteristics of participants, the context in which the work is to take place and the resources available. Planning must include developing preliminary ideas about the:

- philosophy – values of the organisations promoting and doing reminiscence
- people – facilitators and reminiscers
- purpose – objectives of the reminiscence work to be undertaken
- place or space – context and location where it will occur
- programme – what is intended to be covered
- process – what happens during the reminiscence work
- product – tangible outcome(s).

These considerations apply to preparations regardless of whether reminiscence work, including life story work with one person or a number of people, is intended. The list of questions which follows is extensive; it is designed to assist new reminiscence workers and to provide a checklist for those who are more experienced.

The philosophy and values of the reminiscence worker and organisations involved

- Does the reminiscence worker adhere to an explicit ethical code?
- Does the worker understand the ethics, values and ideas which underpin and drive the efforts, including reminiscence work, of the organisations involved?

Guidance

Reminiscence workers who already hold various professional qualifications will be bound by their professions' codes of practice. Others, including self-employed practitioners and volunteers, need to appreciate they are expected to abide by similar values and should ensure that they understand the philosophy and ethical values of any organisation with which they are collaborating.

In all effective reminiscence work, respect for people, regardless of age, culture, ethnicity, gender, sexual orientation, income, politics and religion, is essential. Discriminatory attitudes, conversation and behaviour are unacceptable. Reminiscence workers must model or demonstrate sensitive, anti-discriminatory practice at all times and confidently address any discrimination if it emerges.

Often more than one organisation may be involved in planning and delivering reminiscence. For example a care home may use its own staff to undertake a reminiscence project. Alternatively it may contract with a voluntary community arts organisation to do so or use volunteers either recruited directly or sourced via a volunteer bureau. Unless the overall ideas and ethics of all the organisations involved are compatible and there is general agreement about hoped-for outcomes and ways of working, difficulties and frustrations will arise.

The people involved

- Who and how many people are to be involved as facilitators and participants and why is this number desirable or appropriate?
- Who is likely to benefit from reminiscence and what will best achieve the set objectives?
- Will one person, a couple or small group be chosen and why?

Guidance

It will probably not be possible to work with everyone who may wish to be involved. Choices will have to be made. Individual work is suitable for people who are likely to benefit from undivided personal attention, or lack confidence, or have marked communication difficulties caused by speech, sensory or cognitive impairments. Generally, reminiscence is unlikely to be helpful to people who have experienced serious problems coping in the past and whose present circumstances limit their opportunities for learning new coping skills. Exclude from group work people who are excessively private or socially isolated by personal preference, introverted, seriously depressed, habitually tearful, suspicious, hyperactive, obsessional, markedly agitated, or aggressive. Some people who have such problems may respond well to individual work.

Reminiscence with couples provides opportunities to sustain and strengthen mutually supportive, well-established relationships. Individual work will likely be preferable if there is a known history of marital discord. Group work can provide opportunities for encouraging conversation with people who require speech practice, perhaps following a stroke or neurological impairment. When communication is impaired because of physical or cognitive conditions, it may be easier for people to talk about the familiar past and in so doing opportunities for preserving and transmitting family history may be encouraged.

Small reminiscence groups can multiply such opportunities by also providing social and intellectual stimulation, companionship, mutual support and validation. They can diffuse apprehension associated with more intense one to one relationships. Groups appeal to sociable extroverts, to people wishing to develop new relationships, and to those who like to contribute memories of personal experience to the creation of family histories, public records and accounts of collective history.

The purpose or intended outcomes

- What will be achieved for participants, facilitators and the organisation?
- How can reminiscence work be explained to potential participants and what should it be called?

Guidance

It is important initially to set objectives or anticipated end results regardless of how many people are likely to be involved. Objectives are statements which anticipate outcomes or what it is hoped will be achieved from the reminiscence work. Try to set this out simply and clearly. Any initial statement will probably need to be refined or modified as facilitators discuss it with colleagues and with potential participants. The words used and the name of the group should reflect the objectives and the hoped-for outcomes for both the facilitator and participants.

Application exercises

1. Write down three statements beginning:
At the end of this reminiscence project/group/life story work I would like it to have achieved:

    a.

    b.

    c.

2. An alternative approach would be to write down:
At the end of this reminiscence project/group/life story work I would like the participant(s) to have achieved:

    a.

    b.

    c.

3. Writing competency statements about what you expect you will have learned to do is also common:
At the end of this reminiscence project/group/life story work I shall be able to:

    a.

    b.

    c.

4. Write a simple explanation of the purpose of the project/ group which you could use to invite potential participant(s):
For example: 'I would like to invite you to join a small reminiscence group with six to eight members. We will meet for a couple of hours a week for eight weeks. This will be an opportunity to share memories about the past with each other so that you can value your past experience and discover common interests.'

'I would like to invite you to join a reminiscence group which will...' (complete the sentence(s)).

Leadership and staffing

Reminiscing with only one person or a couple requires only one worker. Any more is likely to be overwhelming. Groups, however, raise a number of more complex questions:

- Who is to lead the group?
- Is there to be one leader or co-leaders?
- What preparation time will the leader(s) have?
- Will the leader(s) have any supervision?
- If so, what will the arrangements be?

Guidance

The number of roles and complex responsibilities in a group justify having more than one leader especially if a worker is inexperienced. In a residential facility or care organisation, decide if the leaders are to be managers or direct care staff or a combination of both. Often a staff member paired with a volunteer brings a welcome blend of familiarity and novelty, of security and new horizons. Adequately trained and supported volunteers contribute immensely providing they feel valued and equipped to fulfil the tasks allocated to them. Whatever combination of personnel is used it is imperative that everyone respects each other and is helped to work comfortably together. Chapter 9 gives more information on co-working or co-leadership.

If a facilitator, especially one with little reminiscence experience, is working single-handed with an individual, couple or small group, adequate time for preparation and opportunities for supervision or review with a knowledgeable person is still important. Such discussion assists skill development and aids reflection about how personal memories and associated emotions are managed when aroused by hearing accounts of other people's experiences.

If leaders or co-leaders are not staff members but come from other organisations they will need to negotiate entry. They must take time to learn about the place in which they will undertake reminiscence work and to meet relevant staff and potential participants.

Co-working is demanding but rewarding. It requires sensitivity and effort to develop trusting relationships founded on mutual confidence and respect. For leaders to compete with each other is disastrous. Roles and responsibilities need to be clearly assigned and may be rotated session by session so that each leader develops a range of skills. There needs to be time outside the actual reminiscence sessions to review or de-brief as well as to plan ahead. This is not a luxury; it is essential for skilled practice. Discussion and reflection with a supervisor gives an opportunity to look very critically at what happened in terms of group dynamics and process, how workers felt, how they reacted and what they might do differently next time. Such stocktaking is not just for trouble-shooting but also for building confidence and skills. Usually the supervisor will be a line manager but it could be someone from outside the workplace such as an independent consultant or mentor who is experienced in reminiscence work.

Evaluation of the whole project, group or life story work once the sessions are completed is also important but is often hard to achieve. Sometimes an independent person who has not been involved in facilitating the work undertakes the task of evaluation. Evaluation means trying to reach a judgement about the worth of the work, considering as far as possible both the tangible and intangible costs and benefits. Inputs, outputs and longer-term outcomes achieved within a defined time period and for whom may be assessed. (See Chapter 16 on evaluation.)

Membership

- Will the group have open or closed membership?
- Who will the group seek to recruit and why?

Guidance

The answers to these questions will influence the objectives set, the style of working and possibly the outcomes achieved. Groups with closed membership are easier to lead than open groups and sometimes there may not be a choice because of the work context. An open group accepts members at any time throughout its existence and is likely to have a fluid membership. The group continues even if the membership fluctuates over time. In open groups members join and leave at any time. This means that members are likely to be at different stages. The development of group identity, trust and cohesion is continually being set back by the newcomers. Longer-standing members may be frustrated and new members may feel like interlopers. In these circumstances relationships can be impeded, work disrupted and members disappointed unless skilfully led by sensitive facilitators.

The context often dictates whether a group will be open or closed. Groups, in assessment units, respite care facilities, acute hospitals or reception centres, for example, where most people remain for only a short time, have by circumstance to be open. A common experience, however, where everyone is facing the same uncertainties associated with illness, crisis, displacement or transition, may compensate to some extent for the difficulties associated with open membership. Groups where members attend intermittently or leave while others remain for the duration and newcomers join at various times are particularly challenging to plan and to lead.

Time-limited closed groups have a fixed number of members who join at the beginning stage, usually within the first two or three sessions, and remain for the agreed duration of the group. Illness, death or other circumstances may mean that some people are occasionally absent or leave for good reasons but in a closed group new members do not replace them. Some groups are very susceptible to losing members. A closed group of frail older people, for example, should recruit sufficient members to ensure its continued viability even if some members leave during its lifetime.

Closed groups move more easily than open groups through the stages from tentative beginnings to established middles to anticipated endings. If handled skilfully by the leaders, these groups give the members a much valued, satisfying experience of group coherence, collective work accomplished, mutual acceptance, intimacy, respect, and a sense of personal and shared achievement.

Group size

- How big should the group be?
- How will this number be achieved?

Guidance
People's ideas about the desirable size of a reminiscence group are very varied. They will partly depend upon the competence, confidence and experience of the group leader or leaders. Groups doing simple reminiscence work are probably best limited to eight to twelve members. More experienced leaders may be able to manage larger groups but these should not be confused with large-scale nostalgic recreational activities like old time sing alongs, retrospective fashion shows, mock weddings, re-enacted fair days or village fetes and suchlike. Participating in these large social events does stimulate recall and can be great fun but is a vastly different experience from the planned small group work advocated here.

Most reminiscence work is best done with far fewer people, and frequently with individuals. Chapter 11 suggests that reminiscence with people with dementia (and some other disabilities) requires very small groups, usually with no more than two to four members along with co-leaders/helpers, and individual work is often more productive than group work. People with hearing, sight or speech problems find it very difficult to participate actively in groups unless special arrangements such as those described in Chapter 13 are possible.

Inexperienced leaders and volunteer reminiscence workers too often allow themselves to be persuaded to work with groups which are far too large to be effective. They risk being overwhelmed from the beginning by an impossible task. Workers should endeavour to develop sufficient confidence to explain the requirements and characteristics of skilled effective reminiscence work and accept that the task of reaching sensible practical arrangements is a vital part of their responsibilities at the planning stage.

Forming a group and inviting potential participants

• Who should decide who is to be invited?

Guidance

Getting a group together requires careful thought and detailed action which various people may wish to influence. Whenever possible, questions about who is to be invited to join a reminiscence group in a residential context should be discussed in staff meetings so that consensus can be achieved. In determining membership it is sometimes helpful to use already existing natural groupings. A key worker, for example, might readily run a group for the residents for whom she has special responsibility. Try to identify other groupings, sometimes called 'natural groups', such as people who live or once lived in the same neighbourhood, town or country, attended the same school or church, worked in the same occupation, had similar sporting interests or shared a common experience such as war service, immigration, bereavement, illness or disability. Select people who are likely to feel comfortable with each other and who will enjoy each other's company, rather than made to feel vulnerable, isolated or embarrassed.

Sometimes the staff may wish to use a group to integrate people, for example a newcomer or an isolated, solitary person. A reminiscence group may then be used to encourage informal mixing in the hope that new relationships will develop. Sometimes the people who reside in one wing of a care home may form a natural group, although the very opposite may work well as the following example shows. According to one care assistant:

> In my home the men and women always sat in different rooms. They seldom mixed with each other, not even in the dining room. We agreed to hold the reminiscence group in the women's lounge and Mr Smith said at the end of the first meeting how much he had enjoyed visiting another part of the Home. He said it was better than having an outing!

Issuing the invitations

• Who should do the inviting?

Guidance

Do not automatically assume that the facilitators are the best people to do this. Frequently they may be but sometimes a key worker or a member of staff who has a special relationship with a person might be better placed. Whoever it is, they must extend a genuine free choice about participation. There are powerful hierarchies in residential establishments and also in other organisations. If senior staff members extend the invitations, some people may feel obliged to accept. Residents may feel coerced while staff members think they are offering freedom of choice.

The format of the invitations

• How are people to be invited?

Guidance

There is no one best way of either selecting or inviting group members. There are many different ways to do both. Choose the way most likely to achieve a positive response. In all contexts, the guiding principle should be open discussion. Sometimes a public invitation on a notice board or a widely distributed flyer works well and avoids accusations of favouritism. Depending on the response, it may then be necessary to think how best to achieve a sensible size and mix of members. If a public invitation is used and more people respond than is manageable, make sure that there will be further opportunities to enable others to participate in the future.

Staff members tend to think they know best who is suitable and unsuitable for reminiscence work. Sometimes they deny opportunities to people, especially those who are different, demanding, diffident or have special needs. Keep an open mind rather than reach hasty decisions. Give people an opportunity to decide for themselves.

It is unwise for inexperienced groupworkers to overload a group with too many people with disabilities. Initially, people may not understand what a reminiscence or memories group means. Some people will be reluctant to try anything that sounds new or strange. These same people may soon want to join, once word has got around that the group is interesting – a resident who first refused an invitation later announced, as she 'squatted' in the reminiscence room, 'I know what you are doing in here and I'm coming!'

For a first group, try to select some natural storytellers or good talkers who will help the discussion along. If the group goes well, confidence will quickly grow, and then in subsequent groups people with more complex needs can be included.

Preliminary interviews

- Is it desirable and advisable to meet potential members individually beforehand?
- Who will do this and how will the arrangements be made?

Guidance

Experience suggests that preparatory interviews are usually important although some workers think they are too time consuming and an unnecessary luxury. Each person, however, who responds to a general invitation to join a group, should be seen before the first meeting if possible. The facilitator can then explain further about the group, gather preliminary background details and inquire what themes or topics the person would like to discuss. This interview should be a two way process. It should give the potential member an opportunity to ask questions to help in deciding whether or not to participate. It should also enable the reminiscence worker to gauge or assess the suitability of the person for the group and what topics are likely to interest them.

A Personal History Form is given in the Appendix to assist collecting preliminary biographical information. This will need to be explained as some people are wary of disclosing personal information to people they do not know well. People are usually ambivalent, if not fearful, about committing themselves to a new experience, so this personal interview acts as a bridge into the group. Be clear about the invitation, sensitive to any reservations or anxieties it arouses, and show genuine respect for the person's hopes and expectations associated with joining the group.

This initial meeting contributes to the 'contract' or 'working agreement' to be negotiated with the whole group during the early meetings, so it is crucial to be able to explain the group in simple, straightforward language. Understanding about the objectives or expected outcomes will grow and develop as the group progresses. This preliminary meeting, however, is vital in securing initial consent and in making the potential member feel that joining the group is a risk worth taking.

Staff members sometimes think that, because they see the potential members every day as they go about their ordinary work, they do not need to take the time to gather initial background information. This is a mistake. Remember that the success of any reminiscence work is closely linked to the attention given to its planning and preparation.

If working with an individual or couple it is also essential for the facilitator to explain intentions, tentatively agree objectives and be explicit about the number, frequency and duration of intended meetings. Be sure to check for feedback from the people involved to clarify any misunderstandings or to identify underlying reservations.

The lifetime of the group

- Will the group be time-limited or open-ended?
- If time-limited, for how long will it last and how many weeks, meetings or sessions will it have?

Guidance

Reaching a decision about the duration of a group depends on balancing expectations, resources and availability of a facilitator and members. Some groups, especially those who see themselves more as local history groups rather than reminiscence groups, are likely to be open-ended and to continue, probably with changing membership, for as long as people wish. They are more like a club or a class and some continue for many years if members are prepared to support them.

It is customary for formed or planned reminiscence groups to meet for a set number of sessions, usually six to twelve. Because it takes a group time to develop and move through the different phases, fewer than six sessions are likely to mean that the group experience will be much more limited and less satisfying than a group which has more time available. Ten to twelve sessions are desirable but be realistic about what can be sustained. Open-ended commitments can be scary whereas explicit time limits can reassure and motivate people to invest concentrated attention and effort.

The frequency of meetings

- How often should the group meet?
- Is the plan realistic?

Guidance

This depends crucially on the objectives or outcomes desired. Once-a-week meetings are conventional but task-centred groups working on a specific project with an intended product may wish to meet more frequently. Groups for people with dementia desirably meet more often than once a week. It is usually better to stick to the agreed number and frequency of sessions rather than let a time-limited group drift on. Finish as planned and then begin preparation for a new group even if it retains some of the members from the previous group. Sometimes groups decide to transform themselves in terms of type of membership and the time span over which they intend to operate, but it is better for this transformation to be explicitly recognised by the group and a new contract agreed. A clear commitment to a set number of sessions increases motivation and heightens expectations. It also assists planning and helps the workers to organise their own workloads.

The place where meetings are held

- Where will the individual sessions or group meetings be located?
- What location is likely to suit the potential participants?

Guidance

Finding suitable accommodation can present many challenges. Make sure the chosen venue will be available for each meeting. People find changes of venue disconcerting. It needs to be accessible, acceptable, well lit, without glare or shadows, comfortable, warm, informally furnished, welcoming, and free from interruptions, distractions or noise. Try not to intrude on other people's 'space', especially if they are not to be included as group members. Such invasions can create resentment. People displaced from their regular sitting areas and favourite chairs may try to assert their territorial rights by gate crashing.

By holding the group in an unfamiliar place such as an underused staff room in a care home a feeling of excitement and adventurousness can be generated. Hospital wards, usually short of small rooms and quiet, private day space, present particular challenges. It is sometimes possible, in spite of obvious distractions, to hold a small group around the bedside of a person who is unable to get up.

Length and timing of meetings

- How long should a meeting or session last?
- What time of day is best for meetings?

Guidance

Meetings vary in length according to the motivation, and the physical and mental fitness of the members. About an hour is usual. Additional time needs to be allowed for gathering together, dispersing and having refreshments. About two hours overall is a rough guide. It obviously takes more time for the group to gather, settle, warm to the work, plan the following session, then to wind down, end the session and disperse than it does for a session with an individual or a couple. Try not to be rushed or to rush others.

Think carefully about the best time of day for holding sessions. This will vary from place to place depending on staff rotas, meal times, other activities, care routines, transport arrangements and preferences of participants. Find a time that causes least hassle for everyone involved and stick to it. For people with a disability extra care may be required to identify an optimum time and location. The agreed time for the agreed number of sessions should be honoured. In these ways workers demonstrate their commitment to the contract and their respect for the work being undertaken.

Escorting

- Who will help the members gather together and disperse?
- If travelling is involved who will be responsible for the arrangements and costs of transport?

Guidance

Be sure to agree an explicit plan about responsibilities if members with impaired mobility require special assistance. Gathering together frail people can be complicated and time-consuming. A co-leader or volunteer may undertake this task or share it with others. Everyone involved will need to understand the importance of timekeeping. Forgetful members will need to be reminded on the day of the meeting and will be helped by having the arrangements written down. Do not ignore transport costs and practical arrangements at the planning stage as they frequently become obstacles to participation.

Seating

- Who will sit next to whom?
- Where will the leader(s) sit?

Guidance

The job of the facilitator is to make it possible for everyone to participate, so think carefully about how the room is arranged, including who occupies each chair. Try to use the accommodation and seating arrangements in whatever ways are most likely to encourage the members to talk to each other, not just to the leader. Think about where members may prefer to sit and which arrangements will be most likely to help them feel secure and confident. Allow extra space for wheelchairs and agree with members where to place zimmers or other mobility aids.

People often try to allay their initial anxiety by sitting next to a friend, spouse or familiar person. As the group develops beyond the beginning stage and confidence grows they may be more prepared to take other seats. It is best to sit anyone who has a visual, speech or hearing difficulty, or who needs special help, near a leader. If there is more than one leader they should not sit together to bolster their own confidence. It is better for leaders and helpers to sit where they can see each other and everyone else so that eye contact is possible and non-verbal communication can be observed. Sitting in a circle or around a table usually works best. Many reminiscence-related activities require a table, which can also provide a sense of security and help people to feel less exposed.

Refreshments

- Will refreshments be served?
- If so, who will be responsible for providing them?
- When will they be served?

Guidance

Refreshments are important to most people, especially those who live alone and who may have few opportunities for socialising. If refreshments are to assist rather than distract, careful planning is required about their suitability, availability, serving arrangements and timing. If served at the beginning of a session they can assist anxious people to relax and to feel welcome. If served at the end they bond people together and may make a meeting very special.

Leaders need to be aware of and make provision for special medical, dietary, religious and cultural requirements and personal preferences. Care home staff will be accustomed to accommodating the dietary requirements of residents, but if not, careful thought will be essential and it may be necessary to seek further information about minority ethnic requirements.

Henley and Schott (2004) advise that many Hindus and Sikhs are vegetarian. Some avoid stimulants, including tea and coffee. Observant Jews and Muslims both avoid all animal products except those derived from animals that have been slaughtered according to religious requirements. Observant Jews avoid milk and milk products within four hours of eating meat or meat products. Shellfish are unacceptable to observant Jews, who may also want to be sure that the cutlery and crockery they use has been kept solely for either milk dishes or meat dishes.

So if people of different religions are involved, it is best to avoid offering shellfish or meat, especially pork or pork products. Animal fat (which, for example, may be contained in shop-bought cakes and biscuits) should also be avoided and vegetarian brands chosen instead.

Always offer a choice of beverages for everyone. As well as tea or coffee, offer herb teas, fruit juice and water. Have disposable cups and plates available for those who might prefer to use them.

Food and its preparation and consumption carry great symbolic and personal significance. It resonates with people's earlier family experiences. Once-familiar food and ways of preparing and serving it, especially taking the preferences and life-time experience into account, can be enormously evocative; its availability can greatly enrich and stimulate the reminiscence process.

Be clear about who is responsible for bringing, serving and paying for the refreshments and clearing them away. If meeting within a residential or hospital facility, try hard to make arrangements that meet the needs and preferences of participants, and the intended programme, rather than the routines of the domestic staff. This may sound a simple task but its achievement can require considerable perseverance and negotiation.

In the words of one care assistant:

> It was after we had turned off the projector, put down the things we had been passing around and the tea arrived that the real chat began. I have never seen the group so animated and excited. I do think it was the refreshments which helped everyone to relax and encouraged them to talk – even Mrs Upta was joining in.

Programme

- What themes or topics will the group discuss?
- How will these themes be organised or arranged?
- What associated prompts, memorabilia and activities will be likely to stimulate memories?
- What other related activities will be used?

Guidance

The choice of themes or topics must rest with the group members. The leader or facilitator will make some suggestions and may propose topics but should defer to the group because, in this democratic style of group work, the group belongs to the members, not the facilitator. Their responsibility is to help the group turn its ideas into a logical and interesting programme that will achieve the agreed objectives. By reading, watching films or videos, visiting museums or accessing historical and local information via Internet resources group leaders can readily familiarise themselves with the broad historical period as well as specific historic events and geographic locations relevant to the life experience and interests of group members (Collins *et al.* 2010). Through such preparation they will be better able to encourage and understand the recalled memories of participants as well as being able to provide appropriate trigger prompts for use in actual reminiscing sessions. Figure 5.1 is a quick reference guide that makes it easy to identify how old a person was at the time of a particular historical event, for example the 1930s depression, the abdication, the end of WWII, the coronation, the advent of the Beatles, the miner's strike or the death of Princess Diana, providing you have an approximate idea of when the person was born.

Born	Age by										
	1900	1910	1920	1930	1940	1950	1960	1970	1980	1990	2000	2010
1900		10	20	30	40	50	60	70	80	90	100	110
1905		5	15	25	35	45	55	65	75	85	95	105
1910			10	20	30	40	50	60	70	80	90	100
1915			5	15	25	35	45	55	65	75	85	95
1920				10	20	30	40	50	60	70	80	90
1925				5	15	25	35	45	55	65	75	85
1930					10	20	30	40	50	60	70	80
1935					5	15	25	35	45	55	65	75
1940						10	20	30	40	50	60	70
1945						5	15	25	35	45	55	65
1950							10	20	30	40	50	60
1955							5	15	25	35	45	55
1960								10	20	30	40	50
1965								5	15	25	35	45
1970									10	20	30	40
1975									5	15	25	35
1980										10	20	30
1985										5	15	25
1990											10	20
1995											5	15
2000												10
2005												5
2010												

Figure 5.1: Quick age guide

Chapter 6 contains examples of some possible themes of interest to people who have spent most of their lives in the United Kingdom. If reminiscing with people from other countries and cultures be alert to the need to check carefully and modify content and triggers appropriately.

Based on the preferences expressed and the information obtained during the preliminary interviews, the worker takes the lead in planning the first session. After that, subsequent sessions need to be planned, at least in broad outline, by the participants, and part of the ending work of each session is to make plans for the following session. It is always important to follow the interests and life experience of the members and to be ready to adapt or modify plans if necessary. Leaders should not impose personal preferences but neither should they abdicate responsibility for assisting the group to develop a coherent programme.

There is no limit to the type or range of subjects to be discussed or related creative activities undertaken. The programme may be thematic or follow a chronological order, dealing with different historical periods, life stages, challenges or interests. Each theme may have within it many different topics, which can be developed over a number of sessions. If a rich vein is opened up, with the group's agreement this can be built on in future sessions. For example: a session on foreign holidays could be followed by sessions on working abroad, favourite foreign food, money and shopping, exotic clothes, music, souvenirs, films, significant buildings, and friends and acquaintances from other countries. One reminiscence worker described how

> I was really interested in the London blitz because my mother had been in it and I wanted the group to talk about that. When I suggested this they said: 'No. None of us was in London during the war. Let's talk about weddings – they are nice and cheerful' and I had to let them.

A similar quick re-orientation was necessary when a worker without prior consultation carefully planned a session on childhood seaside holidays only to have the group members unanimously agree they never went on seaside holidays but always holidayed on the farms of their country relatives.

Process

It is not possible to plan what actually happens with people and between people when they come together to talk about their lifetime experiences. Memories come with accompanying emotions and the skilled facilitator will have sufficient confidence to let the stories be told – even the painful stories and the associated feelings aroused with all their unanticipated surprise and force. Many positive emotions will also be aroused and groups can quickly change from tears to laughter, from pain to pleasure, from regrets to satisfactions. Issues concerned with process are further discussed in Chapter 6.

Triggers or prompts

- Will I need triggers?
- How will all the senses be stimulated?

Guidance

Using multi-sensory triggers or prompts of various kinds to encourage reminiscence is a central aspect of most reminiscence group work. Triggers need to appeal to all the senses of sight, sound, touch, taste and smell because different people respond in different ways. Triggers are especially helpful in the early sessions. Although less common in work with individuals or couples they can also be helpful in speeding up the time needed to arouse interest and achieve warm engagement and mutual sharing of experience. Asking a few simple questions, however, often is sufficient to stimulate effective reminiscence. Most experienced facilitators find that, except perhaps for people with serious cognitive or sensory impairments, triggers are seldom essential but usually extremely helpful.

Locating and using triggers

- How and where can triggers be located?
- How can triggers best be used?

Guidance

Chapter 6 identifies possible multi-sensory triggers relevant to particular themes. It is useful if reminiscence workers or establishments in which regular reminiscence activities occur build up their own small collection of multi-sensory triggers. Collect, beg and borrow objects representing everyday work and domestic life, not grand antiques. Many useful items can be found in junk shops, market stalls, car boot sales and in the attics or cupboards of older relatives. For a small outlay it is easy to pick up second-hand books and magazines, old kitchen gadgets, tools, tins, boxes, cards, coins, clothes, fabrics and household articles. Families, friends and staff are usually very willing to lend or donate things once they understand their potential usefulness.

Music and other sounds are especially good for evoking memories. Recordings of once-familiar sounds such as the whistle from a steam train, children playing, a school bell ringing or the clip-clop of a dray horse can arouse instant recollections. Smells can stimulate memories, particularly those associated with food and home-baking, cleaning, bathing or medicines. For more information about using music in reminiscence work see Chapter 11.

Many people enjoy seeing pictures, projected slides, films, videos, CDs or DVDs. Stories, poems, old newspapers, books, comics and magazines read aloud are very effective. Handling and examining objects, noting their colours, shapes and textures, debating their uses, quite apart from the associated recollections they evoke, can be very enjoyable. Living triggers such as a baby, small child or animal can immediately generate interest, even in the most passive, withdrawn people. Use the natural environment and the seasons of the year. Plants, twigs, bark, leaves, grass, large seeds, pine cones, fruit, vegetables and flowers can all be used. Examples of how to use multi-sensory triggers during the process of reminiscence and life story work are given in Chapter 6.

Libraries, local museums, local historical societies, community groups, churches and mosques, local newspapers and photographic archives are all potential resources. An increasing number of museums are developing outreach services, often based around themed loan boxes which are a way of taking the museum to people unable or unaccustomed to accessing museum services (Group for Education in Museums 2010).

Triggers are readily available once the possibilities in things long taken for granted are realised. Many trigger packages containing tapes, slides and photographs can be bought. These off-the-shelf trigger materials can be useful and, without doubt, they have helped to make reminiscence work popular. The Internet is a huge resource for obtaining visual images and sounds. On the other hand avoid using such resources in a mechanical, routine way because reminiscence work is much more than nostalgic entertainment. It is much better to start with people, not triggers. Discover their interests and concerns first and then look for triggers that closely match. Always begin with the people, not the triggers, unless you use a reminiscence box as an ice breaker and an introductory means of intriguing people and interesting them in the possibilities of exploring further reminiscing.

Equipment

- What equipment will be required?
- What skills are needed to use it?
- What other resources might be needed?

Guidance

Paper of various sizes and colours, pens, markers, card, blue tack, glue and sellotape and access to a photocopier are basic necessities.

Special equipment is not essential but there are times when some can be very useful providing the facilitator feels comfortable with it. If it is intended to use audio recorders, film/slide projectors, video, computers, CDs or DVDs, be sure a competent person knows how to work them. The size of the group will need to be appropriate for whatever equipment is to be used. Inexperienced leaders should always have prior practice with any technology. If co-working, take turns to be responsible for this aspect of a group session as this develops skills and spreads expertise and confidence.

If it is intended to use a projector reduced light may be necessary. An extension lead, table or stand of the required height and either a blank wall, preferably white, or a screen will also be needed. Retain some light if possible and sit people in a semi-circle. Be sure that everyone can see the screen, but bear in mind that low light reduces the possibility of lip reading and the hum of machinery adds to people's hearing problems. Slide projectors are increasingly being replaced by computers, including laptops and digital projectors.

Experimentation with computer software and hardware including touch screens and personalised as well as generic trigger programs is creating exciting new possibilities which promise to make access, storage and retrieval of generic and personal archival and trigger materials much easier (Astell *et al.* 2010). The Computer Interactive Reminiscence Conversation Aid (CIRCA), a touch screen program designed especially for people with dementia, uses generic photographic and video clips to trigger recall. The system is designed to be failure free and to encourage a person with dementia and a carer to enjoy reminiscing together. A second computerised program called 'Living in the Moment' enables people with dementia to engage in interactive artistic activities and games. Other developments such as

PDAs, iPhoto books and social networking sites are opening up new possibilities for computer-assisted reminiscence work. Mulvenna (2010) suggests that computers can be used to support, involve, promote, stimulate, entertain and archive life stories in ways which promote creativity, economy, simplicity, moderation and contextual appropriateness. The increasing acceptability of video conferencing in telehealth care suggests that video conferencing or Skyping could become an effective way of engaging people in reminiscing, either singly or in small groups.

Cameras, especially digital cameras, mobile telephones and home video telephones and conferencing equipment are greatly enhancing reminiscence work (Sherman 2007). Within a year or two mobile phones and devices such as the iPad are tipped to replace laptop computers and are likely to overtake PCs as the most common means of accessing the web. A camera can be used for photographing possible triggers, places and spaces of past or present significance, group sessions and celebrating work undertaken and work achieved. Photography can stimulate 'then and now' discussions and a camera is invaluable for producing material for displays and exhibitions. It is also a great asset in individual life review and life story work. An audio tape recorder for playing and recording sounds, music and recollections is a useful piece of equipment. They vary greatly in type, price and ease of use. Cassette recorders are being increasingly replaced by digital recorders. There is a lot to learn about making good sound recordings but there is no need to be intimidated. Get advice, do some reading and then start practising. (See also Chapter 7.) Recordings of group members' recollections can be used as triggers or reminders or points of departure in subsequent sessions. In this way each group becomes a potential resource for future work. Camcorders offer enhanced possibilities but bear in mind that we have come to expect commercial-quality visual material and amateur film grows less acceptable unless it has particular personal associations.

More people, including older people, are now familiar users of multimedia via the Internet, CD-ROMs, DVDs, email and social networking. These technologies have great potential to stimulate reminiscence, share recollections, locate personally relevant triggers, stimulate recall and link people in new and exciting ways. There continue to be some disadvantaged people, especially older people, who are not computer literate. This may be because they lack the necessary knowledge, have had limited exposure to technology or opportunities for education about its use or lack the confidence to manage any associated problems. It is as well to be alert to these potential problems, all of which can be overcome providing there is an adequate investment of initial time and appropriate training for users – factors which need to be allowed for at any project planning stage.

Before buying any audio/visual or computer equipment, seek independent advice from someone who is technically knowledgeable but who does not have a vested interest in selling a particular brand or product. Make friends with the staff at your local public library. They can assist in innumerable ways. Many libraries, museums and sound archives lend recorders, projectors, cassettes, CDs, DVDs, videos and pictures, as well as printed material. Increasingly many public libraries provide free access to the Internet. Local organisations including libraries, schools and colleges may be willing to transfer video recordings to CD-ROM, computers or possibly MP3s or iPods.

Confidentiality and record keeping

- Are the sessions to be kept confidential?
- Is there to be any feedback and, if so, to whom?
- What records will be kept?
- Who will write them?
- Who will have access to them?
- What will happen to them when the project or group is finished?

Guidance

As part of preparation, leaders will need to have thought about confidentiality and record keeping so that in the first session ground rules can be discussed and agreed. This is an integral part of the contract. The arrangements will vary from project to project, group to group, and between individuals, but it is important that the ethical implications of reminiscence, including record keeping, are always openly agreed and understood. Where reminiscence activity is being used for assisting assessment and care planning this too must be explained.

To be strictly bound by total confidentiality may defeat the purpose of reminiscence work which mostly generates contagious enthusiasm and infectious pleasure. Facilitators and participants may want the mutual enjoyment and satisfaction to be widely communicated. Sometimes, however, in a group when a member has disclosed a very intimate or private recollection, the leader may need to contract with the group about treating that particular episode as confidential. For example a facilitator may say:

> Mrs G. has just trusted us with a very private memory. I suggest we all agree to regard it as confidential and not tell anyone outside the group what we have just been told. What do you think? Is that agreed by us all?

Leaders need to be open about their participation in supervision or consultation. Do not assume that participants understand that staff members may be accountable to line managers for their work. Explain briefly what the arrangements are and what obligations a leader has to colleagues, managers or funders. Assure participants that discussion and analysis of work undertaken is a necessary part of professional development and accountability. Volunteers also must abide by agreed rules and arrangements.

Record forms

- Will special recording forms be used?
- How will these be created and who will complete them?

Guidance

Whether a facilitator is obliged to keep records for supervision or not, it is still an excellent idea to do so because it helps reflection on the work done, week by week, and assists with making an overall final evaluation as well as assisting the development of good practice. Chapter 16 contains further information on record keeping used for the purposes of accountability and evaluation of effectiveness. Examples of various record forms are given in the Appendix.

Agree who is to write any sessional records and who will have access to them. Records should be kept in a safe place. At the very least, keep an attendance record and follow up any absentees week by week. A good way of improving interpersonal skills is to make a 'process' record of any parts of a group or individual session that went either very well or very badly. Try to remember exactly and write down accurately what triggered these 'critical incidents', who said what, the emotions expressed or withheld, and how facilitators and others responded. When a project/group is ended decide what is to be done with the records.

Product

- Who 'owns' any tangible outcomes or products from the group?
- What agreed uses might such products have?
- Who benefits financially from any publications or sales arising from the group's work?

Guidance

It may seem strange to be wondering about 'property rights' and sales before a group has even met. This is, however, another ethical issue to be carefully considered. If the group hopes to publish, exhibit or in some way make a tangible record of its members' recollections, the group will need to agree and to give permission. If life stories, photos, video recordings or personal memorabilia are to be used outside the group, it is a wise precaution to ask members to sign a simple release form at an appropriate time (see Appendix Form 6 for an example). People are seldom reluctant to publish but you must not take agreement for granted. Written permission is very strongly recommended.

Some people find it hard to believe that their lives are worth putting into print or that their experience could possibly interest anyone. Even a modest document produced with a personal computer and photocopier can give its author enormous pleasure, pride and satisfaction. Work that is accessible to other people may have implications for people who were not involved in its creation or even know of its existence. Great care needs to be taken about any possibility of misrepresentation or defamation and it is as well to consult with senior staff and managers to ensure that the requirements of sponsors, host organisations and funders are respected in terms of confidentiality and other ethical issues.

Conclusion

This chapter stresses the need for careful, systematic, detailed preparation. The major decisions required at the planning stage have been identified and general guidance given. Use the chapter as a checklist for planning each new project or group and make brief notes about what you need to do before beginning the first session. Avoid thinking that, because a facilitator has led a previous group, preparations for a new group or project can be skimped; complacency leads to poor practice and unsatisfactory outcomes.

Key points

- Take time over detailed preparation. It will pay off in the long run.
- Select members with great care, usually after a preliminary interview.
- The group belongs to the members, not to the leaders who are enablers, not owners – servants, not masters.
- Do not avoid problems concerned with planning, hoping they will go away. They won't. They will lurk, going underground instead, waiting to sabotage the future work when least expected. So deal with them openly but also learn to be adventurous, prepared to modify arrangements if future circumstances require it.
- Learn to begin with people, not triggers, and to understand what is happening in both intellectual and emotional ways between all involved.
- Build or borrow a collection of relevant multi-sensory triggers if possible.
- Develop the habit of keeping records to help develop the skills required at different phases throughout the life of a reminiscence project or group.

Application exercise

Plan a reminiscence project with a group, couple or individual, using the seven 'P' headings of philosophy, people, purpose, place, programme, process and product to help guide you through the preparation and planning phase.

Further reading

Agrigho, B. (1998) *How to Help Reminiscing Go Well: Principles of Good Practice in Reminiscence Work*. London: Age Exchange.

Doel, M. (2006) *Using Groupwork*. Abingdon: Routledge.

Rainbow, A. (2003) *The Reminiscence Skills Training Handbook*. Bicester: Speechmark.

Chapter 6

Reminiscence Work with Groups – The Beginning, Middle and Ending Phases

Learning outcomes

After studying this chapter facilitators should be able to:

- identify roles, responsibilities and behaviour of workers and members during the beginning, middle and ending phases of a reminiscence group with closed membership
- explain the possibilities and pitfalls associated with using multi-sensory triggers
- differentiate the major characteristics of reminiscence with groups which have either an open or closed membership
- list examples of universal topics or themes.

Beginning phase of a group with closed membership

Although this chapter refers to group work, much of the content is also relevant to reminiscing with individuals and couples, about which more detail is given in the next chapter. Having completed the planning and preparation phase facilitators should now be ready for the group to meet. The first meeting of a new group needs to affirm everyone's best hopes, not confirm their worst fears. Facilitators need to 'tune in' to how they are feeling and try to imagine how the members may be feeling as the first meeting gets under way.

Members will probably be feeling much the same as the leader, both fearful and expectant. They will be ambivalent, torn in two directions at the same time. They will be worried about embarking on a new experience. This is especially so if they have not previously belonged to a formed group, do not know other participants or had previous unhappy experiences in groups. They may also have only a hazy idea of what reminiscence means and what will be expected of them: Will they be able to cope? Will they be pressured into talking when they would prefer to remain silent? Will they be overshadowed, or perhaps overwhelmed, by dominating, talkative people? Will they talk too much themselves or give too much away?

While being fearful, they will be looking forward to a new experience, meeting new people, hearing about new things and wanting to share some of their own past experience and to have it valued and validated by others. If there is more than one leader or helper, tasks should be allocated beforehand so that uncertainties or confusion do not aggravate the ambivalence and tentativeness of members. Ideally facilitators will have met members beforehand but this is not always possible. In order to overcome initial anxiety, be present when people begin to arrive so that each person is greeted by name and feels welcomed and reassured. The leaders have a crucial responsibility to help people feel that the effort they have made to come is appreciated and that they will find the experience worthwhile.

Introductions

At the beginning most people worry about fitting in, of having enough in common not to feel isolated – this may be a major difficulty for people who feel different from other members, perhaps because of language, class or education. Depending on whether or not members already know each other, the leader needs to make introductions. Initial awkwardness can be reduced if informal refreshments are available as people arrive or some memorabilia or photographs are displayed to encourage spontaneous conversation. When it is time to begin the facilitator should encourage people to sit according to a pre-arranged but not rigidly enforced seating plan. Some groups begin by inviting people to introduce themselves. This sometimes works well because it gives everyone an equal chance to participate but it can be very daunting for a shy person to have to speak up in front of everyone right at the beginning of a new group.

Use each person's preferred name – never a name that the leader assumes a right to use. People should be asked what they prefer to be called at the initial interview and their wishes respected. In making introductions, do nothing that might show up anyone's poor memory, or embarrass them in any way. Use name badges with big clear printing.

An alternative way of getting started is for the facilitator to make preliminary explanations and then invite people to pair up with someone they do not know to say who they are and to briefly share two or three pieces of information about themselves. The leader needs to stress people are free to say only what they wish. After five minutes re-form the whole group and in turn let each person introduce their partner to everyone else. Although this is time consuming it is an excellent means of starting to achieve group cohesion.

Contracting

Follow the introductions with a brief statement about why the group is meeting and what is hoped the group will accomplish. This introduction repeats the initial explanation and the tentative contract agreed when first meeting members. If there wasn't the chance to meet people beforehand, the explanation about the group's purpose and objectives must be very clear and the facilitator should 'reach for feedback' to ensure that the members understand, even if tentatively, what they are being invited to do. A simple opening statement from the worker might be:

> We have agreed to meet here today and for ... weeks at ... to talk about past times and to share our memories with each other. Usually people enjoy sharing their recollections about the past. We think we shall all benefit by doing this and today we shall begin by talking about ... Later in today's session we shall make plans for future meetings. Is that all right? Do you have any questions?

Leaders need to clarify what it is hoped the group can offer its members and what the group might accomplish. This contracting work is very important because it makes the members feel that the group genuinely belongs to them. It also means that in future meetings, if anyone wants to use the group for some other purpose, for example planning a fundraising event or advocating with local politicians, the facilitator can return to this agreement or contract. It can then be reviewed and participants can democratically decide if it still represents their wishes, or in what ways it should be changed.

New leaders find it very hard to reach for feedback at the beginning of a new group. This is because they are anxious that the arrangements they have worked hard to put in place at the planning stage might be upset, and plans undermined. Do not be afraid of trusting the group. A group has to be mutually satisfying to be successful. It never will be if leaders insist on imposing their own agenda. Encourage everyone to talk who wishes to express an opinion. Open-ended questions such as 'Is everyone agreeable to this?', 'Is everyone happy with these plans?' or 'Does someone have another idea?' indicate a genuine desire for the group to be founded on mutuality, with everyone sharing and participating as equals.

Ground rules

Some leaders like to agree ground rules at the beginning to try to help a group discipline itself but, if this is done too early or too insensitively, it may make the leader look more like a bossy teacher rather than an enabler or facilitator. This misperception may happen anyway if the leader is already familiar as an authority figure – perhaps as a senior member of staff who is already known as the 'boss'. All groups actually start long before the first meeting to which people bring their prior experience and personal preconceptions so what may seem like a democratic group to a facilitator may not be seen in quite the same way by all the members.

For example:

> Ask the group: 'Do you think it might be helpful if we agreed a few simple rules among ourselves so that everyone gets a chance to join in?' Seek feedback. 'Is that all right?'
>
> Then continue: 'I don't want to sound like a referee but it may help if we agree that everyone who wants to talk should get a chance to do so. Could we agree that only one person speaks at a time so everyone can hear? Is that okay? People are not expected to always agree with each other but I do suggest that we should respect different points of view, and not use unkind or offensive language. We need to accept that old memories might bring up strong feelings. We might get a bit emotional at times. No one needs to feel embarrassed if this happens. We also need to talk about confidentiality. Maybe we should take these points one at a time... What do you think?... Are these suggestions okay?'

It is a mistake to use the first session exclusively for contracting and planning. Although some time must be spent on these aspects, be sure to do some reminiscing in the first meeting so that members leave with a feeling of excitement and a first-hand flavour of what they have come together to do. Otherwise they will be disappointed and puzzled. An opportunity for the group to grow together through shared work will have been lost.

Sessional structure

As already suggested in the previous chapter every session has a beginning, middle and end that should guide the leader's behaviour. So when the introductions and the preliminaries have been completed, introduce the first topic or the first trigger by asking a simple question such as 'What does this remind you of?', 'What does this take you back to?' or 'What comes to mind when you think about...?' Don't rush. Follow the pace and mood of the group. Do not worry if the discussion seems untidy, muddled, irrelevant or disjointed. It usually takes two or three sessions for a group to settle down, for everyone to feel comfortably relaxed, sufficiently confident to initiate discussion or to listen patiently to other people. Keep observing the members continuously to be aware of individual responses. Be finely tuned to the emotions being expressed, not just the words spoken. Reach out to anyone who looks uncomfortable or upset and value everyone's contribution.

Timing

Watch the time. Stick to the agreed arrangements, otherwise some people may be inconvenienced. As the time gets close for ending the session the leader should begin sessional ending work by reminding the members that time is nearly over for today. Briefly summarise what has been done and suggest the group makes plans for its next meeting. Every small detail about all future sessions does not need to be agreed but the broad directions do.

For example:

Say to the group: 'Time is nearly up for today but we still have ... meetings ahead. You remember that we agreed that we might possibly talk about A, B or C. What order do you think we should take these topics in? What would you like to cover in the next meeting?'

If particular tasks or responsibilities need to be allocated agree the details. For example, a member might volunteer to bring a particular trigger to a session or ask a friend or relative for relevant information. After details have been agreed check back.

Ask: 'Is that all right? Are you all happy with these suggestions?'

When the necessary arrangements have been agreed, thank everyone for coming and indicate that today's meeting is over and that it will be good to see everyone again at the next session. People who need to leave can then do so even if others want to linger awhile.

Reminiscence groups often start up again even after such ending work has been done. Do not be worried about this. Animated conversation may also continue outside the session and it may involve others. This does not matter provided that agreements about confidentiality are honoured. Holding a reminiscence group prior to lunch in a day centre, for example, usually results in members energetically continuing to reminisce over lunch; members' enthusiasm is the very best advertisement and is highly infectious.

Group process

Each subsequent session should begin with a modified form of sessional contracting, and end by spending time planning the next meeting. Every group is dynamic – it grows and develops over time. Agreements or contracts are not straitjackets that should never be modified. On the other hand, a group needs coherence, structure and order if it is not to be a free for all, at the mercy of the member with the loudest voice.

Many inexperienced leaders worry about 'losing control'. They imagine that somehow the group will run away from them, people will either talk too much or talk too little and that good order all depends on the leaders. Such worries are diminished if facilitators realise that they are a part of the group and that, although they have special responsibilities, the group belongs to everyone in it, not to the leaders.

People in groups behave differently at different stages. Do be patient. In the beginning phase, most members (and leaders) are anxious. Some people will talk a great deal and appear to be very domineering. This is often a cover for insecurity. Others will retreat into silence and yet resent the seemingly confident talkative members, even though such dominance saves the quieter person from feeling compelled to talk.

In the beginning, members tend to talk more to the leader than to each other. Friends and acquaintances may talk (or whisper) to each other and to people sitting next to them while seeming to ignore, or not be interested in, what other members have to say. People may lack the confidence to talk to the whole group but they relax in time and there are ways of helping everyone feel more comfortable and more willing to contribute. Spending some time in a paired activity and then sharing the outcomes with the whole group can help build confidence in early meetings. Seating arrangements, themes, topics and related activities and how the worker behaves also impede or assist the growth of confidence and mutual trust.

Using triggers in the early sessions can bolster an inexperienced leader's confidence. Triggers, if carefully chosen, quickly arouse interest and encourage conversation. Triggers used in the beginning stage of a group should relate generally to the known life experience of as many of the group members as possible and not be focused on a single member's experience or interests. At this early stage avoid triggers that are likely to relate to potentially intimate, painful or private experience. Topics and triggers should not trap people into too early or too intimate disclosure of potentially emotionally laden memories.

A way to encourage silent or shy group members to participate is to purposely select triggers that relate very closely to their background or interests, if known, and which they quickly recognise and feel knowledgeable about. In this way people may very gently be encouraged to share their memories. People take time to develop trust and respect for each other. Conversation in the early days of a group's life is much more likely to be general, relatively superficial and less likely to involve the sharing of painful, contentious or emotionally charged personal experiences. Increasing self-confidence and willingness to share personally significant memories with other group members will emerge over time when the group has developed trust and intimacy in the middle phase of its work.

Middle phase of a group

After two or three meetings, the group moves into the middle phase. It begins to feel less tentative, surer of what it is doing, safer and more cohesive. During this stage, trust, respect and courtesy emerge. People attend to what others are saying and respect or tolerate divergent points of view. The talkative, dominating member gradually learns to listen and the quiet, retiring member, feeling valued, begins to talk.

Sometimes there may be a few members who cause unease in the group. Monopolisers feel compelled to hold forth, to dominate and to prevent others from speaking. They may have been welcomed at the beginning but increasingly they will irritate other members who are likely to show their disapproval in non-verbal ways. Some people remain aloof or isolated for various reasons although they may very much wish to be fully involved. Feeling rejected by others they may become increasingly hostile, which increases their isolation still further. Some people act the clown, seek attention or compete with other members or with the leader who is responsible for assisting each member to feel comfortable, trusted, secure and valued within the group.

Some members risk becoming a scapegoat if the facilitator is not vigilant. A scapegoat is a person on whom the hostility of the group is projected. Others may recognise in this person the characteristics they like least in themselves. The scapegoat may be an innocent victim but is more likely to have some characteristics that provoke the other members to treat them badly. The leader must actively encourage full participation of all members from the beginning by providing direction and guidance. If such dysfunctional roles still become established, the leader then needs to be able to engage the group and the particular person in discussion about what is happening. By the middle stage, members are more able to discuss such problems openly and suggest solutions. The worker must not take sides but be able to see all sides and to help each member feel able to contribute constructively to the group. Again ground rules can provide a helpful means for ensuring that everyone is listened to and everyone has had equal time and opportunity to participate.

Asking questions

Even the type of questions a facilitator asks can encourage or discourage discussion. Learn through practising to appreciate the difference between open-ended and closed questions. The first invite descriptions and elaboration of memories of events, places, experiences, relationships, things and feelings. The person answering the question decides what to say or not say. The choice is theirs. Closed questions tend to feel like a cross-examination. Save such questions for filling in later details or expanding a story once the discussion sparked by open-ended questions is flowing freely. For example, 'Tell me about your school days' is an easier starting point than 'What was the name of your first teacher?' 'What do you remember about starting work?' is better than 'What kind of clothes did you wear on your first day at work?' Most closed questions require only the briefest answers. Some have yes/no or only right or wrong answers. So if a person lacks confidence or is unable to remember instantly on demand, rather than risk getting the answer wrong, they will probably play safe and say nothing.

Open questions leave control of what is told in the hands of the storyteller and invite responses that others can add to and embroider. Some responses may have various interpretations; some will be metaphorical or symbolic and others literal. Further gentle questioning may be necessary to make sure that everyone understands what is being said or intended.

'Please tell us about your childhood' is likely to produce interesting recollections. 'What sort of food did you like as a child?' will elicit more varied responses than 'Did you like milk?' Such a question could easily be answered by just 'yes' or 'no' although if phrased differently it could prompt an entertaining discussion about school milk, school dinners or other likes and dislikes.

There comes a time when it is appropriate to look for more detail, to encourage people to explore their memories in greater depth and to re-encounter, reconstruct and re-appraise their stories. Throughout the lifetime of a group, leaders and members need to tread softly; everyone has their own pace for developing confidence and empathetic understanding and for earning the privilege of hearing and sharing their own and other people's memories.

Facilitators need to learn to be aware simultaneously of the group as a group and also of all the individual members. They are responsible for the group as a whole and for each separate member. This may seem a tall order but the skills of observation and empathetic response grow with practice (Doel 2006). Having a co-worker greatly assists with keeping track of how each person is responding. Whole body communication is important. Use eye contact, lean towards people to engage them, encourage the silent members to contribute but do not pressure them to do so. One simple trigger, or just a short open-ended question, may be sufficient to start people talking but triggers that stimulate different senses in sequence are powerfully evocative.

As the leader, do not regard yourself as the historical authority. You are an enabler whose task is to encourage the members to talk to each other. They are the authorities and the teachers. If the focus from the outset is on the members' own life experience and personal memories, then obviously they are the experts. The facilitator's responsibility is to help them make connections between their own experience and the experience of other members.

Inexperienced reminiscence workers often use too many triggers. They seem determined to use everything they have prepared, even if discussion is flowing freely. Facilitators need to be orderly and responsive, systematic yet flexible. They need to follow the flow and feelings of the group. Respect the pace, preoccupations and mood of the group as a group, and each separate member. Do not rush or pressure people but also be alert to possible boredom, restlessness or resistance. Sometimes best-laid plans can go astray, as this worker found:

> Because the projector wasn't available we used two large pictures as triggers. One was of a shop and the other of the inside of a country cottage. Although I was worried about having to change my plans and the amount of time ahead, I was pleasantly surprised to find the group members getting great enjoyment from talking about every detail in these pictures. As Mr K. talked I could see a transformation taking place. The members changed from passive observers with very brief comments to excited participants who could not wait to talk about churning, milking and local creameries.

Responding to pain and loss

As time goes on, members will begin risking stories that have layers of meaning. They may try out different versions according to how they 'read' or perceive their present audience. Some may feel sufficiently safe to talk about painful recollections. Others may be reluctant to do so, frightened of their own pain – perhaps fearing being left worse off, rather than better off, as a result of allowing a long buried hurt to resurface or surface for the first time.

Facilitators need to be particularly alert to loss in all its many guises. No one grows old without experiencing repeated loss. This may be of loved ones, family, friends, relations, home, neighbourhood, belongings and pets. There may also be diminished energy, ill-health, moving, enforced or voluntary, from familiar places to new surroundings and lack of once-absorbing interests. As loss encroaches and people face the inevitable comparisons between their past and present circumstances and altered relationships, they may be reluctant to expose their pain. Responding sensitively to any such reluctance or display of hurt becomes part of the reminiscence worker's responsibility. Some members may want to talk while others may be afraid to listen because they fear being overwhelmed by the pain aroused in themselves by hearing other people's recollections.

Many leaders are reluctant to encourage members of reminiscence groups to share pain. In a million ways they damp it down, choke it off and encourage the group to retreat into superficial conversation. The most frequently asked questions by trainee reminiscence workers are 'What will I do if someone becomes upset by recalling sad memories?' or 'Am I doing harm if reminiscence makes someone cry?' Learn to overcome personal reluctance to share another's hurt. Strength lies in being heard. Point the group members towards each other and make links between the members' experience. In uncovering memories, perhaps seldom or never talked about, group members discover common ground and become rich resources for each other. Remember that older group members will probably know more about loss than the younger facilitator does, so use their vulnerability, their resilience and their strength to involve the whole group.

Emotion will never be far from the surface in any reminiscence group. Quickly the mood can change from gaiety to sadness, from laughter to tears. Do not be afraid of tears nor think harm is done if people cry. Tears are seldom harmful. Inevitably some people will recall very painful past experiences. This recall may bring distress or even embarrassment but also relief. It may be the first time such troubling memories have ever been shared. Too often we seek to protect ourselves from pain and upset by fleeing from other people's tears, sadness, disappointment or anger.

Learn to respect silences. Do not be apprehensive nor hurry people on. People need time if they are getting in touch with deeply felt emotions and they need time to organise their thoughts and decide how much they will share. It is not a time for rush or bustle or quick, slick responses. Do not dread silence. Learn to wait out the silence, to name the emotions being expressed and then to link the experience and the emotion of the individual with the experience and feelings of the rest of the group members. The group is the resource. Use it to the full, but be aware that follow-up outside the group may also be necessary if anyone has been greatly distressed by his or her recollections. Very occasionally a person may need expert professional clinical help to resolve recurring, disturbing memories of past trauma. It is the facilitator's responsibility, usually in consultation with mentors or supervisors, to ensure that the person is referred, with their consent, for counselling, psychotherapy or other professional assistance (Hunt, Marshall and Rowlings 1997; van de Kolk 1994).

A few members may never talk or they may talk very little but their body language will indicate how they feel about the group. Silence does not necessarily mean disapproval or lack of satisfaction. Try to understand what the group experience means for each individual and enable them to use the group in whichever way best meets varied personal needs.

When members begin to contribute their own personal triggers this is a sure sign that the group has become important to them. Great sensitivity is needed, however, as some members may no longer have access to cherished possessions. A thoroughly satisfying experience for some members may heighten a sense of loss or isolation for others. Seeing other members contributing personal memorabilia may increase their own feelings of loss, and separation or dislocation from their past lives, unless facilitators encourage them to talk about objects of personal significance even if they are no longer physically accessible to them. In such circumstances it is always possible to suggest to these people that they remember a significant object – seeing it in their mind's eye – and describe it and its significance. In this way they are still able to contribute to the group discussion.

Loss of momentum

During the lifetime of a group, energy and involvement will fluctuate from meeting to meeting and also within meetings. Over time, if members seem to lose interest, do not just silently deplore this, feel hurt or blame yourself. Try to understand what is happening and openly address the issue. Confronting is a very necessary skill in group work but it is one that leaders are often hesitant to use, especially in groups for older or vulnerable people. Confrontation means facing people with the implications of their behaviour that may be preventing the group accomplishing its agreed goals. Confrontation must be accompanied by genuine empathy and concern, not anger or recriminations – otherwise group members will experience the leader as hostile. Confrontation does not mean anger, blame or conflict. It means honestly exploring difficulties, facing up to problems together by having open discussion and jointly agreeing a way forward. Such a process can release new energy as the members re-commit to further work for the duration of the group. See Chapter 7 for further information if it is intended to produce a tangible product.

Absenteeism in formed groups

If the group is a formed group with closed membership and a member is absent, this should be acknowledged in the session. Any absences should be followed up by telephone or visits and explanations or apologies given to other members. Sometimes people change their minds about participating, deciding that reminiscence is not for them. Such views should always be respected but make sure that there is no other hidden reason for a person withdrawing which requires remedial action by the facilitator.

In groups with a predominantly aged membership, intermittent attendance, illness, hospitalisation and deaths are not unexpected. Such events must be openly acknowledged and this will demonstrate to other members that should they experience similar problems they can expect to be treated with equal respect and concern. In care homes good communication with staff members about attendance will be essential if regular participation is to be maintained. Other demands and institutional routines such as bathing, medical treatments, chiropody, hair appointments and unscheduled visitors can all disrupt attendance if communication is poor or staff members do not share the same priorities as the reminiscence worker.

Ending phase of a group

In time-limited groups that meet for an agreed number of sessions, it is usual to foreshadow the end of the group from the beginning. Some weeks before the end members can be reminded of how many sessions remain. In this way the end is openly anticipated. Endings, like beginnings, are a time of increased opportunity for work because they are a time when feelings are more exposed. Groups that have been successful, that have worked well together and shared much, end with less pain than those which have never really 'got going'.

Even in successful groups, members are likely to experience mixed emotions around the ending phase because they will be separating from the leader and from each other. Some may feel relieved that the group is over. Others may resent that it is not continuing, or feel sad or angry that they must face another ending. Leaders may feel pleased with their achievements or possibly guilty because they did not accomplish more. Probably everyone involved will experience a mixture of these varied emotions.

In the ending phase, leaders have a big responsibility to make sure that the ending, with all its mixed emotions, is openly addressed. Do not let a group just fade away, even if some members have anticipated its ending by ceasing to attend. Unfinished business needs to be addressed, achievements reviewed, feelings shared and work evaluated. Use part of the last session for stocktaking. Invite the members to look back, to acknowledge the work they have done together, and to say what the experience has meant.

Try not to be talked into extending the life of the group. There may be considerable pressure to do so – 'just a few more sessions' is a commonly heard request. It is usually wiser to stick to the contract but to be open about how people, leaders included, feel because the group is ending. Facilitators need to be aware of and express their own feelings about the group's ending. If there is a realistic chance that there can be another reminiscence group, say so. Do not make promises which cannot be kept. Common examples of unrealistic promises include promises to continue to visit a facility or visiting people in their own homes. Facing the pain of separation openly is more constructive in the long run than pain denied.

Many groups try to handle their strong feelings around endings by having a farewell party, which tends to emphasise the positives and ignore the pain of impending termination. Of course, there is a place for parties, special events and celebrations but, if these are left until the final session, rich opportunities may be lost for building on a positive experience which is often better situated before the final session. A shared outing or other special event before the last meeting can be relished, recalled and used constructively to promote future recollections. The final meeting can still be special if it reviews, evaluates and celebrates the work accomplished.

If the group has agreed to produce a tangible product such as a publication or exhibition, make sure this is completed. Be clear about the time-scale and mutual responsibilities. On no account promise a product if necessary resources are unavailable.

Endings also mean that the facilitators need to review and evaluate their work. Just as after each session it is important to spend time considering how the session went, so at the end facilitators and helpers should look back to reflect on all the work they and the group have done together. Review the notes from each session. Reconsider what objectives were set and identify what has been accomplished. Try to be realistic. Give credit for work accomplished as well as facing up to the things that could have been done differently, or done better. If effective skilled reminiscence work is to be firmly established it is essential to understand why any project or group has been successful (or unsuccessful) so that next time mistakes can be avoided, skills consolidated and learning implemented. Chapter 16 contains further information about training, staff development and evaluation.

Open groups

In reminiscence groups with open membership, meaning that membership changes from meeting to meeting, group intimacy may never be achieved although participants may still find the experience worthwhile. Each meeting will need to be more or less self-contained because continuity of participants and programme cannot be guaranteed. Leaders need to be very active in such groups which usually have a set programme and often use triggers as a focus for discussion. Such groups commonly aim to provide recreational activities and social and intellectual stimulation; often they are considerably larger than formed groups with closed membership.

As hospital stays shorten, and respite care and intermediate and short-term admissions increase, formed groups with closed membership become more difficult to sustain, except in long-term health and care facilities and community settings. Workers need to take account of the particular context in which the open group is being held and adjust the objectives, programme, process and practice according to the people and place involved. Because it may be impossible to gather initial background information from individuals before they participate in an open reminiscence group, the programme should cover topics of common interest that are likely to appeal to all participants. A skilled facilitator will still be able to achieve positive outcomes but the group is unlikely to develop the same degree of purposeful engagement, trust and intimacy as a closed group.

Men's groups

Reminiscence workers who most frequently are women often suggest that they find it difficult to interest men in reminiscence work. Instead of concluding that men are not interested in recalling and documenting their memories it is wiser to examine the nature of the reminiscing opportunities which are made available and to question whether reminiscence workers are sufficiently responsive to men's needs and interests. Single sex groups, where possible led by male facilitators, may be more acceptable and many examples of successful men's groups have been reported as the following example shows:

> A long established community-based carers' group in reviewing its work identified an increasing absence from its regular meetings of male carers so decided to form a sub-group only for men. In a series of get-togethers, the men discussed issues related to being a male carer but identified another shared interest in local history linked with their own past experience. They agreed to meet with a female reminiscence worker paired with a male creative writing teacher over a number of weeks to explore their memories of work and family life and then to write and proudly publish a small book entitled *Memories... From the Corners of Our Minds*.

This group also illustrated a common observation which suggests that, in introducing reminiscence activities, men tend to be more inclined to begin by talking about work rather than personal relationships whereas women tend to reverse this order. While these gender preferences are unlikely to be universal, nevertheless the choice and timing of themes and topics, and the kind of multi-sensory triggers used initially, as well as the nature of any tangible outcomes or products suggested, requires careful thought. Occupations, education, cars, sports, clothes, conquests, family responsibilities, DIY, health, family history, travel, war service, national service, politics and innumerable other topics, if addressed from a masculine rather than a feminine viewpoint, have all been used to generate fruitful discussions.

Using multi-sensory triggers

Many different approaches are used to stimulate the sharing of memories and to encourage people from varied cultural backgrounds and people with or without disabilities to participate. Facilitators should not assume that what is significant to them will be equally relevant to other people. There are triggers that possibly have universal familiarity whereas many others are likely to be culturally specific. Both verbal and non-verbal communication is important in reminiscence work so that various creative artistic activities are often used as means for prompting recall as well as vehicles for translating or transforming people's memories into visible tangible products or performances.

Some groups like to draw or paint, sometimes accompanied by music, to read aloud, write or recite poems, sing, dance, act, relate stories, complete proverbs, do quizzes, take and organise photographs, make collages, mosaics and wall hangings, do needlework and draw maps, diagrams, family trees and time lines. A list of such possible products is given in Chapter 7. Many such activities are also appropriate when working with individuals and couples. There is no limit to the possibilities, provided people freely agree, feel supported not pressured and no one is made to feel in any way inadequate or demeaned. It is customary to describe multi-sensory triggers or prompts as appealing to the senses of vision, sound, touch, taste and smell. The discussion which follows refers primarily to the general experience of the majority white population of the UK. To appreciate the different experience of immigrants from other countries and cultures that are now growing old in the UK and what might jog their memories, *Mapping Memories: Reminiscence with Minority Ethnic Elders* (Schweitzer 2004) is a valuable source. In the book and accompanying CD Pakistani, Caribbean, African and Asian elders recount their stories and provide information about culturally sensitive triggers and linked creative activities.

Visual triggers

Visual triggers are the most readily available and include pictures or paintings of people, places, things and events. Posters, maps, flags, drawings, diagrams, documents and certificates are all possibilities. Photographs are widely used in reminiscence work but it is important to know that people from some religions and cultures are wary of photographs and some forbid them altogether.

There are three broad types of photographs: personal, artistic and documentary. Look for photographs that combine the personal and the documentary. Even if using a picture of a particular place, one that portrays people and if possible action will be a more effective trigger than a beautiful lifeless scene. The emotional connection stirred by the photograph as much as the photograph itself is important in reminiscence. Use pictures of ordinary people doing ordinary things. Photographs are powerful memory joggers and reveal much about people's personal backgrounds. Pictures of public events, for example the coronation, the assassination of President

Kennedy, Princess Diana's funeral or the twin towers 9/11 disaster, can be used as spring boards for saying to people 'Tell us what you were doing on the day when...' This approach links the public event together with its personal impact. Such events vary enormously in their impact on individuals and may be of little interest or relevance to some people either from Britain or from other parts of the world. Take care if using this approach not to choose events that may make some people feel defensive, uncomfortable or excluded. It may be possible to locate a local public photographic collection or a private collection belonging to someone who has documented community changes over the years. Local newspapers are a good source and amateur photographers are often delighted to discover a 'therapeutic' use for their life-long hobby and willingly lend or permit their pictures to be copied. Museums, libraries, galleries, businesses, schools and colleges can also be good sources.

The digitising of photographic collections makes it easy to store large numbers of images on computer hard drives, memory sticks, MP3s, iPods, CD-ROMs and DVDs. Search facilities make it easy to locate pictures or sets of pictures concerned with specific topics, locations, periods, events or subjects. A laptop computer, screen and data projector enable easy viewing. Enlarging and mounting on laminated card increases a photograph's usefulness and prolongs its life. Several copies of the same picture allow group members to closely examine and discuss pictures with each other. This is a useful technique if people have hearing, sight or speech difficulties.

Newspaper articles and advertisements can be easily enlarged or scanned. Again, having them enlarged, copied, laminated, mounted or put in plastic sleeves extends their life. Colour photocopying produces high quality copies cheaply and quickly. The Internet has transformed the task of obtaining relevant visual and auditory triggers that match or closely relate to the known life experience and places of significance for many individuals, families and communities. Google maps are another resource.

Objects too precious to handle may be photographed. Nothing, however, replaces the sensory intimacy and impact of actually handling an object. Postcards, books and magazines are another source. Local newspapers frequently publish photographs of past times with accompanying articles that are excellent for reading aloud. A reminiscence session may need little more than a local newspaper or an old advertisement to start discussion.

Slides, audiotapes, CDs, DVDs, videos and films need to be used very selectively. They tend to encourage passive rather than active viewing. Historical films should be used cautiously. A few minutes' viewing of selected clips may be sufficient to stimulate discussion. Many programmes made for schools are useful for reminiscence groups of all ages. Any reminiscence aids or triggers must be regarded as servants, not masters. Their purpose is to encourage people to talk with each other, not just to sit passively watching or listening to yet another 'show', entertainment or 'lesson'.

Auditory triggers

Memory for sounds can be vivid and immediate. Often a sound is associated with a visual memory and it may be quite impossible to separate the two. By triggering one, both are evoked. Sounds, especially music, provided people can hear sufficiently well, can be very evocative. Collections of recorded sounds, for example of animals, bird song, trains, whistles, factory hooters, cars, machinery, motor bikes, sea, wind and rain, are readily available. Music of all kinds and periods, songs, bands, film soundtracks, stories, poetry, wise sayings, plays, place names, autobiographies, documentaries and stories recounted in local dialects can be purchased or often borrowed from libraries. Some reminiscence workers like to make their own local recordings and also to use recordings from reminiscence sessions as a resource in later sessions. The poetry archive (www.poetryarchive.org) is an invaluable source. Local radio too is useful as the closer the sounds, content, speech and accents match people's own backgrounds, the richer and faster the response is likely to be.

Music

Music is particularly effective because it immediately arouses emotion. It stimulates while also usually being relaxing, making people feel at ease. It can be enjoyed in its own right and also for the associated memories it triggers. Locate music that reflects varied tastes and experiences. Remember that musical tastes do alter over time so try to discover what music people once enjoyed, now prefer and may now like to hear. Live musical performances by amateur and professional musicians are also very popular especially if the musicians are able to respond to personal requests. Often talent near at hand goes unused. Many older people have retained musical abilities that can be revived and give pleasure to themselves and other people. Procedural memory, including the ability to play musical instruments, can be well preserved. People need to be encouraged and invited to perform. 'It's not my place to put myself forward,' a resident in a care home said with much feeling when the daughter of another resident asked her why she did not volunteer to stand in for a pianist who had failed to arrive for a church service being held in the home.

Provide opportunities for older people to acquire new musical skills and also extend their appreciation of music. Most people can play simple, if unfamiliar, percussion instruments with little instruction. Drumming is particularly worthwhile as a small group activity. Encourage active participation in music making, including choir singing. But beware of making older people feel either patronised or embarrassed. There is a world of difference between recalling or re-enacting childhood experiences and performances and being treated as a child. Recorded music, karaoke tapes, song sheets and large print songbooks can encourage people to venture into active music making.

If using group singing, give all members a chance to suggest a song, even if they are not keen to join in the singing. Some people may have sung in choirs or performed in groups or bands and may gain much pleasure from once again having the opportunity to perform. Respect varied choices remembering that home entertainment such as singing around the piano and listening to the radio or phonograph would only slowly have been replaced by television from the 1950s onwards. Chapter 11 contains more information about linking music and reminiscence work.

Movement and dance

Embodied practices whether dance or movement and connections created between people by means of shared motion, often in a circle or linking by means of balls, scarves, long elastic bands, ribbon sticks, touch, chants, song or other music, can all help people to communicate. 'Dance is a statement of emotion expressed as movement' (Coaten and Warren 2008, p.66). Dance may be a new experience for some people but for others it will be familiar and revive memories of earlier experiences, rusty skills and floods of associated emotional memories about the people, places and times remembered. Even physically frail people with impaired mobility can benefit from chair exercises. Wheelchair dancing for people with various neurological disabilities is possible. Social dance stimulates easy recall of earlier times, significant places and associated relationships in addition to improving balance, being personally affirming and much enjoyed by many people.

Tactile triggers

Pallasmaa quoting Merleau-Ponty's revealing statement, 'touch is the parent of our eyes, ears, nose, and mouth' (2005, p.3), stresses the importance of touch. Handling objects provides instant pleasure and immediate recall. Just holding something, looking at it, feeling its weight, shape and texture, turning it around for closer examination and then passing it to another person links people together in time and place. While being outside the object, in our 'mind's eye' we connect with other times and other places and it becomes easy to share associated memories. Objects also encourage demonstration of how they were used by drawing on long-term procedural memory. They invite activity, opinion sharing and animated conversation. Everyday items like working tools and household gadgets that people can handle easily without fear of damage are preferable. Strange objects whose function is not immediately apparent encourage debate, even disagreement and lively discussion. One day care worker recounts:

> We had a dolly, which is a thing used for washing blankets, but hardly anyone knew what it was for. Someone said it was an ear trumpet. Another person said it was for clearing drains. There were the greatest arguments. Everyone joined in and enjoyed the fun.

Select triggers with care so that over the weeks everyone's life experience can be represented in one way or another; this encourages everyone to feel that their past, and consequently themselves, has been acknowledged and their stories heard.

Tastes and smells as triggers

Even if these senses are dulled by age, tastes and smells can still be used, either alone or combined in sequence with other triggers, to help a group to get acquainted, enrich a theme or explore a topic. It is very easy and inexpensive to assemble a smell collection. Put the same substance into several matching small bottles or containers that can be passed around a group; a lively guessing game spontaneously erupts.

Similar and contrasting smells encourage people to identify, distinguish and name the smells as well as discuss the contexts in which they experienced these odours and the associated memories. Some possible smells include:

- disinfectants and household products – carbolic soap, Jeyes fluid and mothballs
- toiletries – baby powder, lavender water or eau de cologne, after shave, brilliantine and cosmetics
- medicines – menthol, castor oil, eucalyptus oil, petroleum jelly (vaseline) and boric acid
- herbs and spices – mint, chives, rosemary, coffee, cocoa, cinnamon, nutmeg and ginger
- flowers, vegetables and other plants and leaves – lavender, eucalyptus, sweet pea, cabbage, leeks, garlic, spring onions, turnips and potatoes.

Old fashioned sweets and drinks like sherbet, liquorice, jelly babies, 'conversation lozenges', sherbet, and ginger beer can still be purchased and used to stimulate recall. Reminiscing about favourite foods, associated smells, shops and shopping excursions and related people and events can be easily encouraged. Reading old recipe books, recalling food prepared for special occasions, packets, tins, wrappings and advertisements can all be used. Vivid recollections are achieved by actually preparing, serving and eating special food. Cooking old favourites can also involve other staff and relatives in the reminiscence work. Whenever possible, involve all the group members in some aspect of the food preparation, by identifying and demonstrating appropriate tasks or in giving advice and instruction, sharing associated memories and eating the outcomes.

Reminiscence on the theme of food may be a way of reviving dormant cooking skills and rekindling or creating fresh interest in nutrition and personal caring which can be especially useful if people are beginning to pay less attention to these aspects of daily living. One care worker said:

> We were talking in one session about summer time, gardening and fruit picking. This led on to what our mothers used to do with the fruit and we began to talk about making jam. Mrs Smith said how she wished she could still make plum jam and the group then decided they would like to do that, with everyone sharing a part of the job. We got a lot of help

from the kitchen staff but everyone did something to help. We all had such fun. The best part was when everyone had scones for tea and ate our group's plum jam. We were so pleased with ourselves.

A cooperative activity like this could be focused on many other cooking or household tasks such as butter-making, cooking pancakes (perhaps on Shrove Tuesday), making soup or baking bread. It could also incorporate a trip to orchards, farms and farm shops, gardens, farmer's markets or local shops. Polishing silver and brasses, sanding and painting, cleaning and polishing, planting seeds and pricking out seedlings are all possibilities. Almost all activities or actions can call on past learning and if people are so inclined or encouraged can lead on to swapping stories (Craig 2005).

So many reminiscence-linked activities are possible that, instead of listing them here, groupworkers should let their imaginations run free; think of ways of enriching spoken or written stories on the themes below through linked activities or actions. The process once begun will stimulate further recall by reviving other memory systems; storytelling bonds people together and frequently provides great hilarity.

Examples of themes:

- home life
- clothing
- housework
- work
- leisure

- childhood
- school days
- ambitions, hopes and dreams
- wartime
- travel

Any of these themes could be used for several sessions or just for one, depending on the interests of the group, the triggers available and whether the group might like to write or record its recollections. These stories could then be read aloud and used to prompt subsequent sessions. Many of the suggested triggers relate to more than one theme. Each broad theme contains many different topics within it. For example, the theme 'the place where I grew up' can lead to recalling places, times, people, sounds, smells and events. It could also lead to discussion about home as a place which as teenagers we couldn't wait to get away from and in old age we long to return to. Only some of the many possible themes and topics with related multi-sensory triggers are listed. Discover the innumerable possibilities all around and near at hand.

Loan boxes

Many museums, libraries and some community-based organisations and reminiscence centres in the UK and further afield now offer loan box or handling box services. Boxes are a means of making a variety of multi-sensory triggers easily available. Such services also provide a focus for reminiscence training and for promoting and sustaining reminiscence networks consisting of interested people and organisations in local communities.

Usually a loan box service is run on the basis of a time-limited borrowing period, commonly two to three weeks on a collect and return basis. Sometimes a modest deposit or borrowing fee is charged. Boxes tend to be organised around themes. Items are frequently donated in response to public appeals and also by borrowers and users. Most include various small articles such as tools, clothing, toys, books, CDs, newspapers, related annotated photographs, a folder containing an itemised inventory, descriptions and background notes of the contents, brief guidance notes on how to undertake reminiscence work, and evaluation and suggestion sheets.

Some popular box themes include:

- home and family life
- time off and leisure
- rural life
- WWII

- childhood and schooldays
- grooming and fashion
- leaving home
- men at work

Unpacking a box is a journey of discovery for people of all ages and backgrounds which never fails to stimulate animated discussion and give mutual pleasure. The boxes have proved an easy introduction to reminiscence work while readily leading on to further involvement and related creative activities. They have become vehicles for community outreach by assisting unaccustomed users to avail of museum and library services. They can be a source of new acquisitions, archival material and volunteers, a focus for promoting reminiscence networking and, in some communities, encourage community development and greater social inclusion of incomers and marginalised groups.

'This service has given the museum a place in the community' reflects the experience of one education officer whose vision had grown far beyond the long established customary museum work with schools. Her museum through establishing a loan box service had come to embrace a wider involvement with other age groups and community organisations. While greatly contributing to the further development of reminiscence activity, the museum acquired greater knowledge of the local history and involvement in the contemporary needs and aspirations of the community it served. This education officer further commented:

> This loan box service has provided the Heritage and Museum Service with a unique opportunity to engage with a diverse range of people and groups. It has helped to raise the public profile of the Service and has strengthened our links with the wider community. (Edwards 2010, p.28)

Table 6.1: Examples of topics and related triggers	
Topics	**Triggers**
Childhood	
Parents and grandparents	Brandy balls, aniseed, sherbet fountains, liquorice, mint balls, paradise plums, gobstoppers, barley sugar, jelly babies; conkers, skipping rope, dolls, dinky and matchbox cars, board games, mecano, lego, mechanical toys, teddy bears, marbles, comics, club badges, cigarette cards.
Brothers and sisters	
My favourite toy	
My favourite place	
Rhymes, songs and riddles	
Street games and pastimes	
Toys, books and comics	
What you did on a wet day	
How you spent Sunday	
Visiting the sweet shop	
What parents' jobs were, paid and unpaid	
Taking care of younger children	
Clothes you used to wear	
Rewards and punishments	
Surprises and disappointments	
Doing odd jobs and messages	
Pocket money and how you spent it	

Table 6.1 *cont.*	
School days	
Journey to school School buildings, classrooms and playgrounds First day at school Learning to read and write Teachers, liked and disliked What I kept in my pencil case What I kept in my desk School dinners and free milk Lunchtime and break time Playground games, sports and trouble Truanting, mitching, bunking off or missing school Best friends, gangs and secret places My proudest and most embarrassing school events Special occasions, speech day, sports day, concerts and plays Leaving school School reunions Going to college	Slate and pencil, chalk, reading book, copy book, exercise book, crayons, wall chart, maps, jotters, ink, ink-well, nib, pen, fountain pen, biro, text books, school photographs, school clothes and uniforms, school satchel, haversacks, books, bags, badges, school bell, roll call, reciting tables, reading poems and stories, singing, school reports, programmes from speech days and sports days
Home life	
The street where I lived The house where I grew up Bathing and hair-washing Meeting people and making friends Courtship and marriage – 'In my day...' 'Young ones now...'	Photographs, autograph books, postcards, maps, carbide lamp, torch, safety razor, shaving brush, shaving mug, nutmeg and grater, snuff, paraffin lamp, Jeyes fluid, mothballs, carbolic soap, shroud and bed linen, Vicks chest rub, camphor, cookery books, cards, curling tongs,

Weddings	pre-decimal money, photograph albums, Christmas cards and decorations, flowers, plants, seed packets, seed catalogues, gardening tools and mail order catalogues.
Setting up house	
Pregnancy and childbirth	
Illness, home remedies and cures	
Death and funerals	
Family celebrations – Christmas and other festivals	
Favourite food	
Recipes and cooking	
Shops and shopping	
Friends and neighbours	
Clothing	
Changing fashions	Button hook, buttons, hat pins, corsets and stays, braces, hats, gloves, shoes, scarves, boots, shoe polish, lavender, mothballs, cosmetics, perfumes, jewellery, furs, apron, collar stud, tie pin, hats, shoe last, spats, stick-on soles, thread, sewing and knitting patterns, knitting or darning wool, needles and patterns.
Children's clothes	
Teen gear and hair styles	
Working clothes	
Best clothes	
Handing down and making do	
Home dressmaking	
Housework	
Domestic routines	Wash tub and board, dolly, knob of blue, wooden and plastic pegs, Sunlight soap, flat iron, gas iron, electric iron, crockery, bottles, sugar tongs, household linen, starch, feather duster, clothing, knitting needles, sock needles, darning needles, electrical appliances, sewing machine, cooking utensils, kitchen equipment.
Child minding	
Caring for others	
Household appliances	
Wash day	
Starching and ironing	
Going to the launderette	
Drying clothes	
Mending, darning and sewing	
Shopping	
Food and cooking	
Improvising toys	

Table 6.1 *cont.*	
Wartime	
World War I and II – impact on families The day WWII was declared and ended Evacuation and returning home Women's war work, munitions factories and land army Rationing of food, clothing, furniture and petrol Americans and other servicemen Life in the armed forces Air raids and air raid shelters, fire watching and ARP wardens Keeping the home fires burning – civilian and voluntary work Wartime romances Men returning home from the services	Films and books, pictures, paintings, reading war poetry, letters and diaries, evacuation instructions, warden's helmet and arm band, ration book and coupons, identity card, service uniforms, medals, maps, gas mask, recordings of Gracie Fields, Vera Lynn and other wartime music like 'The White Cliffs of Dover'.
Work	
My first job and how I got it My first pay packet and how I spent it Mates at work Pay and working conditions Strikes, lockouts and industrial unrest Being unemployed Trying new directions Travelling to work Leaving home, going into digs Emigrating to seek work Rural work and town work Being apprenticed Domestic service	Pay packet, lunch tin or box, advertisements, train and bus tickets, union card, job advertisements, horseshoe, ears of wheat, corn, barley, hops, tools, working clothes, photographs of mates and works outings, tools.

Shop and office work	
Giving up work to raise a family	
Experiencing retirement	
Leisure	
Going on day trips and holidays	Cinema ticket, chocolate box, ice cream wrapper, concert programmes, postcards, holiday snaps, bathing suits, beer mats, matchboxes, sand, shells, sporting equipment, bus, train or tram tickets, recordings of rock or jazz musicians, for example Elvis Presley, souvenirs and holiday brochures or posters and clips from favourite films.
A day at the seaside	
Trips to the country	
Staying with relatives	
Cinema, music hall and theatre, film stars	
Dancing and dance bands	
Games and sporting events	
Hobbies and pastimes	
Pet animals and birds	
Evenings at the pub or club	
Day at the beach, races, dog track	
Public transport, bicycles, cars and motor bikes	
Package holidays and foreign travel	

Conclusion

Ambivalence is common during the beginning stage of a group while trust, intimacy and significant and sometimes painful memories emerge in the middle stage when important work is accomplished. The ending phase requires skilled leadership and celebration of work accomplished and memories shared. Many themes and topics are available for exploration. It is very unlikely that available subjects will ever be exhausted although varied ways and means will be needed to evoke people's memories. Using multi-sensory triggers will encourage people to share their life experiences. Make full use of the natural environment, people's own possessions and special and ordinary triggers. Museums and public libraries, and specialist reminiscence centres, some with loan box services, are immensely valuable and trips, visits and outings to favourite places can all be much enriched if linked reminiscence is encouraged.

Key points

- The beginning and ending phases of a group are times of heightened emotions and opportunities for significant work.
- It is important to learn to listen to people's memories of loss, pain and sadness as well as to their joys, achievements and humdrum everyday experiences.
- As a facilitator only promise what can be delivered and make sure what is promised is delivered.
- Triggers that appeal to all the senses in turn encourage rich recollections and lively discussion.
- Start with people, discover what might interest them and then locate relevant triggers.
- Develop the confidence to use the rich potential of information and communication technology without forgoing the immense value of immediate stimulation provided by sight, sound, touch, taste and smell accessed by direct interaction with the real world.

Application exercises

Undertake these exercises either on your own or with a potential co-worker:

1. Write a detailed work plan for running a session of a group, listing preparations you will need to make for a possible theme or topic and what triggers you would like to use. Identify any related activities and possible tangible products or outcomes.

2. Run the group session you have planned.

3. After the group session is finished, write a short closing statement summing up achievements for the group and for the leader(s):

    a. 'The group achieved...'

    b. 'I [we] learned to...'

    c. 'I [we] need to continue to work on...'

Further reading

Crimmens, P. (1997) *Storymaking and Creative Groupwork with Older People*. London: Jessica Kingsley Publishers.

Haight, B.K. and Gibson, F. (2005) *Burnside's Working with Older People: Group Process and Techniques*. Boston: Jones and Bartlett.

Osborn, C. (1993) *The Reminiscence Handbook: Ideas for Creative Activities with Older People*. London: Age Exchange.

Sim, R. (1997) *Reminiscence: Social and Creative Activities with Older People in Care*. Bicester: Winslow Press.

Chapter 7

Reminiscence, Life Review and Life Story Work with Individuals and Couples

Learning outcomes

After studying this chapter you should be able to:

- understand the difference between spontaneous or opportunistic reminiscence and prompted or planned reminiscence
- undertake simple reminiscence, life story work and structured life review with individuals
- distinguish between reminiscence, guided autobiographical writing, structured life review and life story work techniques
- appreciate the importance of non-verbal communication and stimulating all the senses
- use various techniques for recording and portraying people's memories
- appreciate relevant ethical considerations.

Reminiscence work with individuals is often referred to as life story work or as life history. In this chapter the words are used interchangeably unless particular distinctions are made. Autobiographical writing and structured life review, two well-researched interventions, will be described in detail. Reminiscence work and oral history also share many common features that are identified in Chapter 8. Much of this present chapter is also relevant to reminiscing with people who have various disabilities such as dementia, depression or impaired hearing, sight or speech, people with learning disabilities and people approaching the end stage of life.

Spontaneous reminiscence

From time to time everyone experiences spontaneous, apparently unprompted recall of memories. Whether these memories are 'entertained' privately or shared publicly with other people depends on personality, circumstances, capacity, motivation and opportunity. This recall may be a fleeting experience or a whole series of linked memories. Sharing these recollections with another person enriches and extends the recall process. Carers in residential facilities, day centres and in domiciliary care as well as volunteers and family carers need to appreciate the importance of encouraging rather than discouraging such spontaneous reminiscence. Many seen and unseen events prompt such memories – an unexpected sound, a whiff of perfume or after shave, children playing in the street, an animal outside the window or a particular taste or tune.

Such unexpected memories surprise us; they catch us unawares and leave our past experience exposed. Vision may confirm what sound, touch or smell has already revealed. When this happens spontaneously it is important to respond with interest, ask an open-ended question that encourages the teller to follow the memory trail exposed and continue the exploration if the person wants to do so. Try to understand what the memory recalled means to the other person, both its significance in the past at the time it was laid down and what it means now in the present circumstances.

In caring situations there are many opportunities to respond positively to such spontaneous reminiscence. It is not always necessary to be 'sitting comfortably' to reminisce. Often a carer may be bathing someone, dressing a wound, making a bed, tidying a bedroom or helping a person to dress or to eat. When these unprompted opportunities arise, seize the moment – it may not come again.

Planned reminiscence with individuals

In addition to these casual opportunities, planned or prompted reminiscence work with an individual can be very valuable. It may be undertaken for many of the same reasons suggested in Chapter 4 but carefully consider why individual rather than group work is preferable. As in group work, the facilitator must be able to explain what is intended and why and to reach an agreement or contract with the person concerned who must have a genuine free choice about participating and understand it is possible to withdraw at any time.

Individual work also needs careful preparation. All the same questions about why, when, where and how need to be considered. Individual work, just as group work, may vary in terms of objectives, methods and outcomes depending on the contract agreed and the skill of the worker. Memory and imagination interact through the process of reminiscence to help us construct a life story or life script that each person can live with. The story locates us within our family and within a wider community and public context. It provides a sense of continuity by helping individuals to appreciate who they are, where they have come from and where they are going. The life story connects the present and the past and gives perspective to the struggle between hope and pessimism, integrity and despair as older people confront the future (Erikson 1982).

As Meip Gies (2010), the Dutch woman who hid Anne Frank and her family during the Nazi occupation of Amsterdam in WWII, said on her 100th birthday: 'The past is never over. The past is always with you. You can learn from the past.'

Getting started

Inexperienced workers often worry about the beginning phase of work with an individual. They ask themselves questions such as: How will I get a shy, reticent person to start reminiscing? Will I be intruding on their privacy? Why would they want to talk to me? A number of techniques can help. One way to start simple reminiscence might be for the reminiscence worker to suggest taking an imaginary walk together down the street where someone grew up. Get the person to describe what is there and talk about both the place and its people. Together it may be interesting to draw a plan or diagram from memory and then name the various landmarks, streets and buildings. It then becomes very natural to describe in more detail the associated memories, people and events tied to these locations. This idea can be developed further by asking about the house in which the person lived as a child – its appearance, sounds and smells – and beginning to walk together, in imagination, through each of the rooms, recalling what each was used for, how it was furnished and any associated special events. People can be asked to imagine the cupboard in which they kept their toys or their clothes, a shelf in their kitchen, garage or greenhouse, and then to talk about and, better still, to demonstrate linked happenings. Depending on their interests, they could be asked about friends at school, members of a sports club or team, mates at work or members of their family.

Some people respond to the suggestion that they should imagine their life as if it were a garden, a house or a party and then to fill in the details from memory. Once begun, the recollections usually flow. The relationship made with any individual person is as important as the memories recalled. This grows out of purposeful work, a shared journey based on mutual respect. Warmth, acceptance, concern and genuineness are the ingredients required if people are to entrust their life story to reminiscence workers.

Using triggers with individuals

Many of the suggestions about using multi-sensory triggers with groups can be applied to work with individuals. Consider the person, objectives, relevance and appropriateness of what is being planned. Enlarged personal photographs are very useful but do not forget other kinds of triggers, especially things that can be touched and handled, smelt or tasted. It is helpful if an individual's preferred sensory pathway can be discovered to guide the choice of triggers. Listen carefully to what people say. The phrase 'I feel...' gives a hint, for as Pallasmaa (2005, p.13) suggests 'the eyes of the skin' are more important than vision which is usually ranked as being the primary pathway to knowledge and memory. 'I see...', 'I think...' and 'I hear...' are phrases that give useful clues about how people process information – their preferred or dominant sensory pathways – and therefore what types of sensory triggers might be most helpful in prompting memories. This pinpointing of a particular pathway is especially useful when encouraging people with sensory disabilities, dementia or depression to reminisce.

Be alert to using a person's own triggers if they are available. This is obviously easier if the person is living at home where there are likely to be all kinds of memorabilia. If they are living away from home, relatives and friends may be able to locate triggers. Follow the interests and preoccupations of the person, trying hard to obtain triggers that relate closely to their known life experience, but failing that use generic objects, pictures and sounds as substitutes.

Making a tangible product

Think carefully about whether it is possible to work towards making a record or a tangible product. Explain some of the different ways this could be done. Individual work may consist only of shared conversation. Sometimes, however, it may be very natural to suggest that a permanent record is made of these conversations. Never impose this on a reluctant person. Be sensitive to any tendency for people to devalue their experience, dismissing their life story as being of no interest to anyone else, and therefore not worth preserving. Women frequently dismiss the importance of their life experience and may need considerable encouragement to start life story work. 'It's not worth writing down', 'I was only a housewife' and 'I never did anything very interesting' are common initial responses. If a permanent record, no matter how modest, is produced, it may be kept only as a private document or be shared with others. Either way it can be of immense value to its owner in terms of preserving identity and enhancing self-esteem. If shared, it becomes an effective tool for ongoing communication with potential to become a valued family legacy. Various formats for making and displaying records are described later in this chapter.

Life review, autobiographical writing and life story work

There are many different ways of doing specific or focused work with individuals. Only some will be mentioned while similarities and differences between life review, simple reminiscence, life story work and guided autobiographical writing will be described.

Evaluative life review

Life review is the kind of reminiscence that has a large element of stocktaking or self-evaluation, of taking a second look and coming to terms with life, however it has turned out. Although still based on recalling and talking about the past, it is more deliberate, systematic, reflective or considered and it results in seeing or understanding the past in a new way. Butler (1995, p.17) stressed this aspect: 'Reminiscence has a constructive purpose... The life review should be recognized as a necessary and healthy process in daily life as well as a useful tool in the mental health care of older people.' Butler suggested that people benefit from the opportunity to express their thoughts and feelings to someone willing to listen. This encourages them to reflect upon their lives so as to resolve, reorganise and reintegrate what may be troubling or preoccupying them. It is generally accepted that interest in 'putting one's life in order' intensifies in old age although many adolescents also struggle with similar issues of identity and self-esteem. A life review can be triggered spontaneously when people of any age are faced with events or crises that confront them with questions about their own identity and the meanings they attach to life. Incapacity, illness or accident, life threatening conditions, bereavement, broken relationships, unemployment, loss of financial security, bankruptcy, moving into care or moving in with a family member, diminished independence, crises of many kinds, both public and private, local, national and international, and awareness of growing old and the inevitability of death can precipitate such stocktaking.

Thinking, remembering, daydreaming and autobiographical, and sometimes creative, writing are all kinds of social interaction with oneself, even if no immediate audience is involved. Having an audience, however, either as listener, reader or viewer, does seem to help to develop a 'good story'. This means a story that makes sense of life's experience, not necessarily a story with a happy ending, but one that represents a person's life in a way that is acceptable to the teller. People may achieve this by working alone – for example when they write a memoir or an autobiography. It seems to help, however, in producing a coherent story, a personally acceptable account, if there is interaction between the teller and a listener, so that the reminiscence worker fulfilling this role makes a considerable contribution.

Structured life review

Although some writers still use the term 'life review' loosely to refer to aspects of reminiscence either with individuals or groups that contain an evaluative element, it is increasingly being used in a stricter, more technical sense. Haight (1998, p.86), a nurse educator and researcher, defined it as:

> A short-term structured reminiscing intervention conducted on a one-to-one basis with an older person. The person who conducts the process acts as a therapeutic listener who guides the older individual in his or her memories, and helps that individual to reframe troubled events and to move on in their thinking.

Reminiscence, guided autobiographical writing and life review have both common and separate characteristics.

A structured life review:

- is undertaken with individuals, including those with depression, and is used selectively with people with dementia
- is a planned purposeful intervention to which the person consents
- usually relies on verbal questions, not on multi-sensory triggers
- is evaluative in emphasis – the meanings or interpretations attributed to the events recounted are more important than the events themselves
- is therapeutic in intention – to help the person come to terms with his or her life
- is time-limited with an agreed number of sessions, usually eight weekly, one-hour sessions undertaken in private. The number and frequency of sessions may be adapted
- is designed to cover the whole life span from birth to the present
- is structured so as to be a chronological or a thematic account
- is a systematic process based on a tested research-based format.

The life review worker:

- guides the person to consider questions concerned with death, grief, fear, religion, school, hardships, sex, work and relationships
- assists the person to analyse troubled events, to achieve their integration and to move on
- uses reflective counselling skills and for this limited time the worker becomes a trusted confidant
- may use Haight's Life Review and Experiencing Form (LREF) to guide the interview (see Haight and Haight 2007)
- uses measures of depression, life satisfaction, communication and cognition where appropriate before and after the life review to assess changes over time
- frequently but not invariably produces a tangible taped, written, visual record or an illustrated life story book
- may undertake a parallel but separate review with a spouse or partner.

Distinguishing characteristics of reminiscence and life review

Reminiscence may be undertaken with either individuals or small groups and can be used with people either with or without dementia of any age. Although planned, reminiscence does not necessarily systematically cover the whole life span but may explore a particular time, period, event, theme or topic. Reminiscence frequently utilises multi-sensory triggers to promote recall. It is not deliberately therapeutic in intention – but may turn out to be so. It is not necessarily evaluative or integrative, although aspects of the process may be because it fulfils various personal, social and cultural functions. Reminiscence may be limited to a fixed number of sessions or be open-ended while its content is not usually tightly structured or rigidly systematic. The worker is an enabler or facilitator, not a counsellor, although the worker seeks to be responsive and reactive and will be prepared to explore feelings and meanings to some extent. Frequently reminiscence will use various creative means to record and present tangible outcomes of the process. Often spouses, partners or other people may share in the reminiscence process.

Guided autobiographical writing

'Guided autobiography is a method of assisting individuals in preparing their personal histories. This process uses life themes and memory-priming questions to help group participants recall and organize their memories' (Birren 2006, p.5). This method assists people to formulate a map for their life's journey to guide them from the past to the present and to face the future with hope arising from confidence that grows as they re-visit their journey thus far.

Birren and his colleagues developed this approach which blends individual work and group work. It involves individuals writing on agreed themes and then sharing their writing with others in a small group where each person reads his or her writing to the other members. Each theme is first discussed in the group in preparation for the writing which takes place in private. The method combines personal recall and reflection with support in a mutual aid group as a means of promoting self-acceptance, insight, emotional development and growth and social opportunities (Birren and Cochran 2001).

In guided autobiographical writing:

- usually ten weekly small group meetings of approximately six to ten members take place. Sometimes up to 30 members might participate in the general preparatory session before dividing into smaller groups
- this structure can be readily adapted, for example to a weekend workshop format
- in private, in between sessions, each person prepares a short two-page written story about the agreed aspects of life
- group members then read and discuss their writing in the group meeting
- group members provide feedback, support and confirmation that life has been worthwhile
- this approach has a sound research base and groups are facilitated by leaders with professional expertise
- it appeals to people who are socially confident and reasonably educated and is a particularly fruitful way of forming new relationships at a time in life when other significant relationships may be lost.

Birren's original nine chronological aspects that can be altered according to particular needs and context in order are:

1. History of the major branching points in life or the time and nature of important decisions
2. Family history
3. Career or major lifework
4. The role of money in life
5. Health and body image
6. Loves and hates
7. Sexual identity, sexual roles and experience
8. Experiences of and ideas about death, dying and other losses
9. Influences, beliefs and values that provide meaning in life.

Selection of participants
Birren and Deutchman (2005) stress the need for careful prior selection of members of autobiographical groups, because it is rarely desirable or advisable to exclude a group member once he or she

has joined a group. They advise against including anyone who is likely to:

- dominate the discussion
- go off on tangents
- not want to write two pages each week
- be shy or reticent and slow the discussion
- make negative or judgemental comments
- pose as an expert on every topic
- speak when others are speaking
- withdraw from the group, looking displeased
- share very serious material at an early session before the group has developed trust
- want to behave as a therapist.

Research outcomes from guided autobiographical writing groups

Research studies reported by Birren and Birren (1996) identify the outcomes listed below for individuals participating in these groups. Participants experience:

- a sense of increased personal power and importance
- recognition of past problem-solving strategies and their application to current needs, problems and anxieties
- reconciliation with the past and resolution of past resentments and negative feelings
- resurgence of interest in past activities or hobbies
- development of friendships with other group members
- greater sense of meaning in life
- ability to face the inevitability of death with a feeling that one has contributed to the world.

Other creative expressions of life review

Similar individual, group or mixed approaches that combine verbal reminiscing and non-verbal forms of expression such as painting and drawing to illustrate different aspects of life experience are also growing in popularity (see also Chapter 15 on end of life issues). Important elements of life may be represented in innumerable ways.

Stories may be illustrated with simple drawings and diagrams. Spontaneous or rehearsed drama, mime, dance and music can involve people of all ages actively re-presenting, reworking, re-integrating and reconstructing aspects of their personal pasts. Many poetry and creative writing groups have a distinctly biographical, retrospective emphasis where the choice of topic may either be suggested by a facilitator or else left to the free choice of each group member. Such writing frequently has a life course focus without being as tightly structured or as comprehensive and deliberately evaluative as either individual structured life review or guided autobiographical writing groups. Brian Keenan (2009, p.264), the Beirut hostage, suggests in his autobiography: 'the past is like an accordion player's moving hands pulling out and squeezing back the melody of memory'.

Life review linked to guided autobiographical writing is also consistent with three-stage recovery models used with people who have experienced traumatic events of varying degrees. Stage one seeks to establish physical and emotional safety. Stage two provides a safe place in which the story of the trauma can be remembered, talked about, mourned and re structured so as to affirm the dignity and value of the person. Stage three provides opportunities for reconnection and engagement in relationships and activities which move the person towards regaining pleasure, well-being and life satisfaction.

Guided autobiography groups that encourage people to write privately as a means of organising their thoughts and rehearsing what will be shared provide opportunities for remembering and mourning, while sharing the story with accepting others brings new understanding of meanings and perceptions, validation and realisation of commonality, at least of some aspects of life experience, and provides opportunities for developing new relationships and renewed social engagement.

Using life stories to illuminate present behaviour

Whether working with individuals or small groups in all caring contexts there will be some people whose behaviour presents challenges to carers and reminiscence workers because everyone communicates through their behaviour. Some people may be excessively demanding and hard to please, noisy, aggressive, hostile, uncooperative and unhappy. Others may be equally challenging because they remain aloof, isolated and negative; they seem to be either unwilling or unable to join in the life around them. Remember that all behaviour has a purpose, even if the purpose may be hard to understand. The meaning behind problematic behaviour is not always easy to fathom and is likely to need some unravelling. Everyone has a personal style formed by the interplay between inherited genetic factors (stability), lifetime experience and more recent or present circumstances (plasticity). Some people may have unrecognised physical pain or discomfort, some may need concentrated personal attention, and others may be grieving for multiple losses, lonely, demoralised or depressed. Lifetime experience, current circumstances and present needs will all influence present behaviour (Jones and Miesen 2004).

Frequently a detailed knowledge of a person's life story coupled with precise observation provides clues to why they are as they are now and some of this information can be gathered through reminiscence and life review. If the person's unhappiness and troubling behaviour can be reduced because of this greater understanding, the quality of life for this person as well as everyone around them can be improved.

Too often staff members attach labels. They 'give a dog a bad name' and then are surprised that the person behaves in exactly the ways expected. Try to pay particular attention to troubling and troubled people. Observe these individuals closely, spend time with them, listen if possible to their life stories or gather life history details from other informants. Consider whether it could be possible that the way that other people relate to the troubled person is in some ways responsible for the present behaviour. When words fail, behaviour becomes a substitute, and carers must learn to 'read' this non-verbal way of communicating instead of implying that the whole responsibility for so-called 'challenging behaviour' rests with the individual who is so labelled.

The more that is known about a person's past, the easier it becomes to understand why they are as they are in the present. This means that carers must take time to listen, to discover – probably from various sources – about their past and then to use the understanding to reach the person in the present (Hubbard *et al.* 2002). Work hard to create situations where the person truly feels 'heard' and respected as a unique individual.

Some people may have been very badly hurt, whether in the distant past or the more recent past. They may be reluctant to talk. It may take time for them to develop sufficient trust to do so. Some probably never will. A key worker system in care homes makes it more likely for warm, caring, trusting relationships to blossom and to establish effective communication.

Many attitudes, approaches and routines encourage difficult behaviour because they serve the purposes of the staff or the institution more than the needs of the residents; they are not person-centred. Some routines are so long-established that no one actually knows any more why certain things are done in certain ways, other than that they always have been!

Try to discover whether behaviour that is experienced as difficult is caused by the myriad ways in which staff members, and possibly family members too, convey their disregard, the routines they impose, or whether it springs from unresolved past pain or unmet present personal needs, including physical pain or discomfort. A careful assessment, combined with close observation, will help unearth possible causes and suggest solutions. Any responses will need to be put into practice on a trial basis because it may never be possible to fully unravel the causes of the behaviour. Both personal and environmental factors that interact with each other will probably be implicated.

Being in care is a sort of bereavement, an awful painful loss, and the resulting grief can be very difficult both for the person and for others around them. Being in care may also revive earlier attachment anxieties or memories of past loss and grief, emotions that are then re-experienced in the present as fresh abandonment (Bruce 1998).

A few people tell the same story over and over again. It is very hard not to lose patience with them. This 'obsessive' reminiscence seems to offer little satisfaction to either teller or hearer. It becomes a recitation of past negative experiences – of 'keeping old sores alive' – that the person seems neither able to accept nor to forget. Reminiscence is not helpful to such people if they are unable, after a time, to move on from dwelling on such memories. They may respond better to other activities that distract them from their preoccupations or to cognitive behavioural counselling through which they may learn techniques that encourage more positive thinking.

Generally, however, whenever people recounting their life stories are carefully listened to by someone prepared to follow wherever the story leads, this will prove to be constructive. The listener must be open to hearing the story, skilled in reading non-verbal behaviour, while at the same time being responsive to the details of the story about the past and to the present emotions that the storyteller is now experiencing as part of the retelling. One care assistant said:

> It was as well that I was there when Tom Jones started to talk about his time as an air raid warden and how he had not been able to get a child out of a building. I listened very carefully and I then asked him about other times and he was able to tell me how he had helped bring out a whole family in a later raid. I do think it helped him not to get stuck just on what he had not been able to do. I helped him see the other side of things as well, to remember times where he had succeeded, and not to blame himself as much as when he first began.

Recording, preserving and representing reminiscence and life story work

There are innumerable ways in which the outcomes of reminiscence with individuals, couples or groups can be represented in tangible formats. Getting from 'process' to 'product', however, requires thoughtful preparation. Time, commitment, talent and resources will all influence decisions about what to do and how to do it. Producing any tangible reminiscence product is demanding for all involved. The production process, therefore, must promise to be enjoyable, and the desired outcome achievable and satisfying. The wish to leave a tangible record behind motivates many people. For some a product is evidence of keeping faith with those already dead. For some it is satisfying proof of the continuing ability to complete a defined task. It may be a means of attaining increased personal understanding and validation, and a way of raising public awareness of times past and lives lived.

Products vary from simple to complex; some are short-lived, others durable; some are created for personal satisfaction, others for public consumption; some require few financial and human resources; others require a complex mix of skills and assistance from many people.

Any envisaged product must be within the resources and competence of participants and leaders to deliver within a realistic agreed time span; otherwise there will be disappointment, recriminations and sapping of motivation likely to overshadow any subsequent project. Attention to the points listed below will help achieve success:

- take time over the planning
- agree explicit allocation of roles and responsibilities which value each person's contribution
- identify and access any required additional expertise
- distinguish the various separate stages to be worked through from conception, through execution to completion.

Many of the approaches described briefly below provide rich possibilities for involving colleagues, family members and friends as active participants, partners and contributors. The process itself, as much as the outcomes, enlivens caring and enriches relationships. Producing a tangible product must always remain less important than the reminiscence relationship and communication on which it is founded. It is well to remember that, while involving family members in reminiscence work can be mutually enjoyable and rewarding, some may discover, perhaps for the first time, aspects of their family history they find deeply disturbing. This can mean that what and how memories are to be publicly represented involves careful exploration and sensitive negotiation. Table 7.1 lists some of the many possibilities, many of which combine performance, visual and written aspects. A more detailed description of a small number of products follows.

Table 7.1: Tangible representations of group, couples' and individuals' personal memories		
Performance	**Visual**	**Written**
Audio recording	CD-ROM	Archive
Charades and mime	Ceramics	Assisted autobiography
Choir	Collage	Biography
Computer networking	Cushion cover	Blogs
Cooking	DVD	Book
Copper working	Display	Diary
Dance	Drawing, diagram or chart	Letter
Drama or brief enactment	Eco map	Life story book
Excursions and outings	Embroidery and tapestry	Magazine or newspaper article
Gardening	Exhibition	Memoir or autobiography
Movement	Family tree or time line	Play
Musical composition	Genogram	Poetry
Musical show	Installation	Postcard
Reading aloud	Jigsaw	School report
Recitation	Life story book	Scrapbook
Singing	Map	Short story
Song writing	Memory box	Spiritual autobiography
Storytelling	Model	
Theatre	Mosaic	
Trip, visit or pilgrimage	Multimedia presentation	
Walking or heritage trail	Mural	
Woodwork and modelling	Painting	
	Papier-mâché	
	Photograph album or display	
	Portrait	
	Pottery	

Table 7.1 *cont.*		
	Quilt	
	Quiz	
	Quotations	
	Rug making	
	Sampler	
	Sculpture	
	Stained glass	
	Story board	
	Video diary or video portrait	
	Wall hanging	
	Wood carving or whittling	

Life story work

Life story work is suitable for people of all ages. It originated in the form of life story books prepared with looked after children who had experienced multiple moves and disrupted parenting (Rees 2009; Rose and Philpot 2005, Ryan and Walker 2003). Life story books or more generally life story work is now recognised as an invaluable tool in care provision for other groups of varying ages, especially, but not only, people of any age who have a learning disability or dementia or are contending with a life threatening illness, who may be living either in their own homes or in care homes. It is also being used successfully with people with functional mental illness, including depression and acquired brain injury. It may also contribute to rehabilitation programmes. Life story work is a loose term which describes how reminiscence is used to encourage people to reflect upon their lives both chronologically and thematically, usually with another person or less frequently in a small group, and then to prepare a 'book' in which written recollections, photographs and any other available memorabilia are included.

Various 'this is your life' type formats are used. A number of commercial products or templates and various online formats are available although the flexibility and economy afforded by a loose leaf binder in which plastic sleeves and pouches are added as required has much to recommend it. The Northern Health and Social Care Trust's *My Life Story Book and Guidelines* (2009) is an example of an attractively produced yet flexible working tool. It has been designed to encourage staff from a number of programmes of care serving different client groups to undertake life story work (NHSCT 2009) with the primary objectives of improving service users' well-being and self-esteem.

Life story work is at the heart of person-in-relationship centred care. Some care homes for older people ask new residents to bring such a personal record with them at the time of admission in order to help staff to get to know them, to begin to make relationships and to aid communication. The book is used to introduce the newcomer and assist settling in. Other care homes make the preparation of a life story book an integral part of a key worker's relationship building in the early days following admission. Such books also serve as 'passports' should a person need to be admitted to hospital or transferred to another facility or as family legacies when a person dies.

There is no standard way of either preparing or presenting a record of a person's life. Some outcomes of life story work are presented in very simple formats, others are more elaborate. It is best to compile the record in ways that make it easy for alterations or additions to be made. This enables personal writing, tape transcriptions, photographs, significant personal documents such as school reports, birth, death and marriage certificates, invitations, letters, personal papers, newspaper cuttings and pictures, and other materials about the person and the period and places in which they have lived to be included. Issues of consent, ownership, access, disclosure and confidentiality are very important and must be negotiated with each person who is asked to work on creating such a record.

A life story book should be a living or dynamic document, a record in progress, not a completed static product. It is subject to change, modification and expansion as its owner continues to reflect upon their life's journey. The process of preparing it is much more important than the final outcome. It is a record of the past as well as a record for the present. It can be updated from time to time but the story is never fully told. Even after a person dies, he or she lives on in the memories of others, exerting an important present influence although physically absent. (For additional information see also Chapters 14 and 15.) Life story work has wide relevance to many people. A care worker in a supported housing facility valued it because 'it has given me a better understanding of some of the problems that many of my elderly tenants have to face' while another commented 'it made me look back on my own life and how I would like things done in the future'. For a son its value was threefold because his 'mother thoroughly enjoyed the experience; we appreciated the additional staff time and their increased personal attention Mum received; and the family is delighted in the new information unearthed and now preserved for us'. A care home manager commented that the book was 'an invaluable tool in that it contains the resident's life history at the flick of a page and this could be used to stimulate conversation'.

Guidelines

- Remember life story work is meant to be enjoyable – it is neither an exam nor an inquisition.

- It is usually undertaken in a series of spaced joint conversations taking account of a person's health, mood and energy levels which may fluctuate from week to week; informed consent or assent needs to be obtained early in the process, not necessarily in the first session, and it should be made clear that a person may withdraw at any time.

- Completion of written consent towards the end is highly recommended. This should cover issues of who may have access to the book, where it will be kept and who is to become its future custodian.

- Respect that the book belongs to the subject person.

- Explain to family members or next of kin, if appropriate the purpose of the book. Seek their cooperation and allay any anxieties.

- If using a template do not use it as a straitjacket but as a flexible guide.

- Agree mutual roles and responsibilities especially concerning the preparation of written material.

- Photographs and documents are better copied rather than including originals.

- Never take over tasks the interviewee might wish to do themselves.
- Wherever possible use the person's own words and capture the emotions attached to the memories.
- Be sensitive to the possibility that significant relationships do not always involve conventional heterosexual marriage.
- Some recollections are bound to be sad and they too will require sensitive empathetic listening.
- Respect any information the person does not wish to have included although they may still have benefited by talking about such recollections.
- Try to go beyond mere facts and encourage reflection on the values that have underpinned the person's life.
- Encourage reflection about how the person sees their whole life and reinforce positive achievements.
- Always seek agreement at the end by working through the book and making any requested alterations or deletions.

Customarily, the conversations on which a life story book is based as well as the contents included are treated as confidential unless the owner agrees otherwise. Life story workers, however, must abide by the policies and practices of their organisations and the ethical codes or guidelines of their professions. If information that may have potential legal or criminal implications is divulged, however, guidance should be sought from line managers, trade unions or professional associations.

Photograph albums

Photo albums with or without explanatory notes can involve a life story approach. Usually photographs are arranged in chronological order over all or sometimes chronologically within themes. Some minimal identification and annotation adds immensely to their present as well as longer-term interest. Careful selection is usually required given the plethora of unidentified family photographs many individuals and families amass throughout their lives. A further development is talking photo albums that readily allow ten seconds of audio recording matched to 24 6" × 4" photos compiled in a battery-powered wallet. The pictures and recordings can be changed as many times as wanted. (See www.talkingproducts.co.uk/talking_photo_albums.htm.)

Family trees

These create a sense of continuity by visually locating the subject person in time and to some extent place. They may also be incorporated within a life story book. Various computer software programs can assist the compilation of family trees although they are not hard to draw by hand. A family tree can be photocopied and enlarged for display in people's rooms in residential facilities. Sensitivity is needed when gathering information to compile a family tree because people may have unconventional families or little known family antecedents that they find problematic to represent in a diagram or may not wish to publicly display. Always seek agreement for whatever is proposed, and do not proceed without consent. Life maps and network diagrams are similar but are fuller diagrammatic representations that contain short explanations about significant events, places and people.

Time lines

Time lines focus attention, stimulate recall and help both teller and listener to keep track of what is being recounted because 'we have a mental need to grasp that we are rooted in the continuity of time' (Pallasmaa 2005, p.32). Space and time are closely intertwined in memory. A time line is a simple chronologically structured way of recording major milestones and significant life events. Time lines are sometimes drawn by dividing them into decades and plotting the important event either above or below the horizontal line to indicate either a positive or negative experience. Sometimes small illustrative photographs are added. If people wish to do so, it is easy to add to a personal time line a parallel time line in a different colour showing major national or international events which help place the personal history within a broader public perspective, and vice versa. Time lines are a helpful introductory training tool for nursing and care staff new to such work. They require exploration with the person whose life they summarise and usually a family informant, which helps to individualise the person and locate present behaviour and circumstances within a lifetime perspective. The carer can be encouraged to undertake a similar exploration on their own account to make themselves more aware of the impact such a journey into the past evokes.

Eco maps

These encourage children or adults of any age to situate themselves within a web of relationships through drawing a series of concentric circles, locating the informant within the central circle and inviting them to situate significant and less significant people in the outer circles in terms of how important that person is in the life of the informant. Eco maps focus on strength of regard or emotional bonds rather than on geographic proximity or distance. Making a drawing such as this is an easier way for some people to talk about their relationships and life experiences.

Memory boxes

A reminiscence loan box contains a collection of memorabilia designed for use by many different people, whereas a memory box contains items owned by or relevant to a specific individual. Many different kinds of boxes have been used as receptacles for these personal collections. Shoeboxes, small suitcases, tool boxes, work baskets and fancy commercial boxes are easily acquired. Any available receptacle that allows for the safe storage of small but personally precious artefacts can be used. Sometimes a memory box is compiled much as an individual's life story book is prepared with the assistance of a reminiscence worker. Sometimes such work is very effective when undertaken as a group project where general discussion takes place first and then each individual works on their own box either at home or in the company of a group of other people similarly engaged. A memory box represents an individual's memories, not a group's collective recall, although people often value meeting in groups with each person being assisted by a reminiscence facilitator or volunteer. Such projects have great potential for including other family members or younger people engaged in intergenerational reminiscence projects. If group sessions are held there will usually be some group reminiscence about universal themes to stimulate cumulative reminiscence. A topic such as 'the place where I grew up', for example, might be discussed together with sharing ideas about how the individual work might proceed. Each person is then paired with a worker or volunteer who encourages the person to think about the choices they might make and do make about the contents of their own box. In later sessions individuals display their boxes to the group and explain the significance of the choices made. This celebrates and validates each person's life while also stimulating further reminiscences.

Public exposure of boxes is not essential and the techniques used vary according to the objectives and context in which the work is taking place. Sometimes boxes are private repositories of personally significant memorabilia compiled to safeguard threatened family history and they are invested with intensely personal memories. A South African example comes from a KwaZulu-Natal project where reminiscence workers assisted families in which parents are dying from HIV/AIDS to record family history tapes and collect memorabilia which are stored in boxes to serve as legacies for their surviving children (Denis and Makiwane 2003). In this project copies of tapes are archived in the local university to ensure the records survive the ravages of time, the death of parents and possible dispersal of other family members.

Another example of a memory box project is the one funded by the European Union and undertaken by the European Reminiscence Network to mark the 60th anniversary of the end of World War II. It involved over 100 elders in seven European countries in which groups of older citizens worked with artists and facilitators to create individual memory boxes out of redundant artillery boxes which served as miniature display cases. 'The elders had the opportunity to reflect upon their past lives with the artists and to explore ways of expressing their memories and their feelings in a powerful visual form' (Schweitzer and Trilling 2005, p.4). The resulting exhibition is still available to tour if funded by a host organisation and can be used by museums, libraries, community arts centres and health and social care agencies as a focus for reminiscence workshops, conferences and visits by groups of all ages.

Wall hangings, collages, quilts, cushion covers, mosaics and murals

All of these may be either individual or group representations of themes, places and people. Usually their preparation runs in parallel with the reminiscing that informs the content, and their preparation involves considerable discussion and effort over an extended period of time. Handwork, however, also is undertaken by individuals working independently as illustrated by the table cover worked in cross stitch and the accompanying book, video, radio broadcast and website created by Jean Baggot – 'an ordinary young girl from the Black Country growing up in extraordinary times'. *The Girl on the Wall: One Life's Rich Tapestry* shows how she merged personal experiences and contemporary public crises by depicting these intertwining experiences as 73 'circles of life'. Completing the tapestry became a passion which led her on to new found confidence and successful completion of a university degree in history, thus making up for the opportunities denied in her childhood because in the prevailing view of the time 'girls didn't need an education because they would work for a short time, marry young and have a family' (Baggot 2009).

Story boards

These provide a visual summary of the major events in an individual's life story gathered by means of reminiscing and consulting other available informants and sources of information. Usually incorporating photographs, they have been used by the bedsides of people in care homes and hospitals and are especially helpful to staff if people are admitted for short-term respite care. Payne (2010) developed a similar but different approach with nursing home residents. He posted summary sheets containing abbreviated life history details gathered from personal interviews outside the doors of residents' rooms as a device for changing staff attitudes by helping them to individualise the residents. Both story boards and summary sheets have great potential in nursing at home and domiciliary care, particularly where a number of professionals or care workers, friends and visitors are involved in providing care. If the person concerned attends a day centre or sheltered workshop this is an ideal opportunity to gather the reminiscences or life story details needed to provide the information in an accessible format. Whether displayed in a person's own home or elsewhere in clear large type with attractive pictures, such displays become a source of information, a focus for communication and a tangible direct reminder of the individuality of the person. Scrap books or annotated photograph albums or life story books may be more portable and can be used in similar ways.

Audio recordings

Audio recording remains popular in both group and individual reminiscence work. Experience shows that it is much easier to make a good quality audio recording of an individual than of a group.

Transcribing an audio recording, although a time-consuming task, increases its usefulness. It provides an accurate record of the story told as well as being an excellent learning tool for critically appraising the skills of the interviewer. The record enables the worker and supervisor or mentor to analyse and reflect upon the interview and to think about alternative approaches that might have been used. Parts of recordings can also be used as links between reminiscence sessions or as triggers to stimulate further reminiscing. Even with a full transcription – a very time-consuming task – an index or summary is very helpful. Usually a copy of the recording and sometimes a transcript is given to the person interviewed.

Tape recorders are easy to use and most interviewees quickly accept them. Very few people find them intrusive beyond the first few minutes of a session. Cassette tape deteriorates over time unless kept in an even temperature and increasingly cassette recorders are being replaced by digital recorders known as solid state recorders which use memory cards for downloading to computers and transferring to CDs or DVDs or external hard discs for long-term storage or archiving. Digital recording technology is subject to rapid development and it is wise to seek expert advice before purchasing any recording equipment. Helpful advice is available from the Oral History Society website (www.ohs.org.uk) about equipment, recording techniques, copyright issues and ethics.

If intending to record an interview, before beginning a clear agreement about what is intended is essential. There needs to be clarity about ownership, access, how and when the record may be used and where it is to be stored. Any reservations about access and use must be respected. A signed consent form is strongly recommended and an example is given in the Appendix.

Reading a simple guide to audio recorders and recording is time well spent. Either poor quality recorders or poor recording techniques produce unusable recordings. Many of the pitfalls can be readily overcome with some simple instruction and practice. Many libraries, local radio stations, museums with sound archives and local history societies are so interested in obtaining oral recordings that they will often lend or hire recording equipment. In return, tapes or CDs will be stored in proper archival conditions, preventing deterioration, and the donor will be given a copy.

Guidelines for making audio recordings

- Use the best equipment available.
- Digital recorders and transcription software is increasingly available.
- Use an external microphone if possible rather than relying on an in-built one.
- If using cassettes C60 or C90 cassettes are more robust.
- Choose a quiet place without background noise, preferably a room with soft furnishings.
- Learn to work the recorder before beginning the actual recording.
- Check and adjust sound and volume levels.
- Place the recorder within approximately 18–24 inches of the person. Better still, use a lapel microphone when recording an individual.
- Use a multidirectional microphone or multiple microphones for recording groups.
- If using a microphone on a stand, do not place it on the same surface as the recorder.
- Plan the interview or group session with care. Have a list of prepared questions to use as a guide.
- Learn to ask only one question at a time and do not interrupt.
- Ask different types of questions including questions about feelings related to the reminiscences.
- Write and also record identifying details giving name, location and date on the cassette or CD and also on its box.
- Keep an index of topics or a summary written as soon as possible after the interview.

Video recording

The same ethical and procedural points already listed also apply to video recording. As video cameras and camcorders have become smaller and less intrusive their usefulness in reminiscence work has greatly increased. Editing software now makes it much easier to produce video films of reasonable quality with less intrusive equipment and less expenditure of time and effort. Remember that it is much more intimidating to be filmed than to undertake an audio recording. Remember too that high-quality television to which we are all accustomed means that poor-quality amateur video film is unattractive and practically unusable.

Although there will be some exceptions, a person talking to camera or to a visible interviewer for more than a few minutes soon becomes rather boring unless action or movement are incorporated or illustrative still photographs inserted. For a time-limited project it may be possible to obtain technical assistance from media studies students from local colleges but this will require considerable preparation during which the purpose, methods, content and outcomes of the project are clarified and agreed by all involved. Video clips have become more versatile and accessible since they can now be so easily incorporated into PowerPoint multimedia presentations for viewing on computers, CDs and DVDs.

Using computer technology for producing life stories
Increasing numbers of people of all ages are now computer literate and the opportunities for acquiring information technology skills and access to computers is steadily growing. Nevertheless too many ageing people still lack these skills and strenuous efforts are needed to spread computer literacy. For the growing number of people who do use PCs, however, there are limitless opportunities for transforming their recollections into attractive, accessible permanent publications or presentations. Many people use email and the Internet to share reminiscences, life histories and memoirs across national and generational boundaries (Aldridge 2003). Provided older learners have access to support as they learn and are highly motivated to persevere with tasks that are important to them, like writing their family history or life story, they are quite capable of acquiring computer skills. They are likely to need more patient instruction, substantial encouragement, reassurance about eventual mastery and considerable practice initially which means they will take longer to learn than younger people (Sherman 2008a, 2008b).

When introducing older learners to computers, the following guidelines are important:

- A relaxed, informal teaching style is essential to allay computer anxiety.
- Provision of copious encouragement, especially in the early stages, until confidence is established.

- Computers need to be demystified and technical language used sparingly and mostly in response to students' questions.
- Being in a class with younger people is uncomfortable for self-conscious older learners until basic computer competence has been achieved. Mixed age groups are then more acceptable and often helpful and enjoyable.
- In the early stage of learning, twice-weekly sessions are recommended.
- Ready access to a computer for additional practice in between sessions is desirable.
- Open learning manuals or notes enable each student to work at their own pace.
- A non-competitive, cooperative, sociable learning environment encourages older students.
- Motivation is increased by early and frequent evidence of achievement in the form of hard copy or PowerPoint presentations.
- Informal assistance from older mentors is most acceptable and much appreciated.
- A club rather than a classroom ethos has wide appeal and increases motivation.

Teaching older people to be responsible for their own writing and its production in an attractive format which can include scanned or digitised photographs and other material has limitless possibilities. Acquiring computer skills and using them to accomplish reminiscence and life story work, or other tasks of personal significance, is experienced as genuinely empowering.

Some people are content to write for their own private consumption; many write for the benefit of their families. Others are driven by a desire to publish. Writing is a complex time-consuming process and its success depends on a number of factors. These include:

- present circumstances
- the intensity of emotion associated with the original memories and their recent recall
- the effects of rehearsal on the intensity and the detail of the reminiscences recalled

- the need to reconstruct memories so they fit with the writer's present ideas about themselves, how they wish to be perceived by others, and the meanings they now attach to their lives.

What people record, write and make public encourages others to begin to write. Much autobiographical writing occurs in private without the validating response of other people, as occurs in a guided autobiographical writing group. The Internet with its opportunities for social networking and blogging using sites like Twitter, Facebook, Be bo and innumerable others has opened up access to a virtual audience for exchanging memories via chat rooms. It also provides a ready outlet for people to create their own home pages, to share their life stories and publicise their creative writing (Sampson 2004).

Reminiscence using the Internet as a means for linking frail and isolated people as well as being a source for locating reminiscence triggers has many possibilities which health care workers seeking to achieve health gain are beginning to use (Collins *et al.* 2010). Using US IN2L technology, Fold Housing Association's 'Brain Bus' provides accessible on-site opportunities for people with dementia to use the technology to access a wide range of relevant visual and auditory prompts. The equipment which is mediated by attendant staff is used to spark conversation, promote social interaction, reminiscence and recall and play games. A large screen linked to a comfortable modified exercise bike allows users, if so inclined, to combine physical and cognitive exercise by cycling through a bespoke virtual landscape depicting familiar personally significant landscapes and locations from the individual's past or present experience. The technology can also prompt reminiscence and enable personal recollections to be logged, stored and printed as hard copy suitable for cumulative compilation of life story books as well as providing information relevant to assessment and care planning (see www.brainbus.co.uk).

Microsoft PowerPoint life story presentations using CDs and DVDs

The major motivation for compiling multimedia presentations of life histories is the wish to leave behind a record, most often for the benefit of the family. Related purposes are the achievement of greater personal understanding through life review and the attainment of wisdom. These same formats can also be used to access relevant personal triggers to stimulate autobiographical memories and promote conversation with people whose memories are being compromised by dementia or brain injury. PowerPoint can be readily used to compile CDs of a person's life history. The various stages of doing this include selection and scanning of photographs, recording and matching digital audio files of spoken reminiscence and music and creating and copying the CD. Desirably the photographs and matched sound recordings should represent the person throughout their entire life from earliest childhood to the present.

Recordings may be made in private but more and richer memories are likely to be evoked if the stories are recounted to one or more people. A digital audio recording requires a computer with a sound card, a microphone connected to the sound card and editing software. PowerPoint enables text, photographs and recorded audio and video clips to be incorporated into a single presentation. The presentation then resembles a slide show with commentary viewed on a computer screen or projected onto a larger screen by a data projector with speakers. Hyperlinks permit quick access to slides so that it is easy to move, say, from a set of pictures of childhood to a set portraying adult life or sets of pictures of different locations lived in at various stages of life.

Digital storage means that multiple copies of a CD can easily be made possible for each family member. If writable DVDs are used instead of CDs increased storage capacity will enable several members of a family, for instance, to store their presentations on a single disc. The use of a DVD drive will enable presentations, not necessarily in PowerPoint, to be displayed on a television screen using a DVD player which dispenses with the need for viewers to have a home computer.

Not everyone will wish to undertake the whole production process. Once having assembled the photographs and audio and video recordings, in itself a worthwhile undertaking, a person may prefer to hand over the technical aspects of production. Such facilitation and partnerships make excellent intergenerational projects that link older and younger people together, but the leaders need to have had adequate training in reminiscence work in order adequately to prepare and assist the participants. If older people are helped to learn and use the ICT skills required this greatly enriches their satisfaction and self-esteem. Attention to the process, including sensitive attention to the associated feelings aroused in the recall process, is pre-eminent, although the objective is the desire to create a tangible product for personal, family or wider consumption.

Increasingly 'life historians' are offering similar services on a commercial or social enterprise basis. Storycorp is a fascinating large US project whose website accessed at www.storycorp.com describes how the organisation encourages older people, accompanied by a younger relative, to record and archive their life stories. Starting from the simple invitation 'Tell me about your life' many thousands of Americans have now recorded and archived their life stories for the enrichment of their families and themselves.

Ethical considerations

Reminiscence work with individuals, couples and groups raises a number of ethical concerns. Autonomy, choice, consent, respect for difference and ownership of outcomes have already been mentioned. Issues of fairness, benefit and risk are also relevant. Fairness means that each person engaged in a project has equal or acceptable opportunity to participate and contribute according to their capacity, motivation and needs. The reminiscence experience should not harm but rather benefit all the participants in the careful judgement of the worker. One of the biggest threats to the well-being of people living in institutions of all kinds, especially older frailer people – and also to many elders living in the community – which is seldom taken into account, is the risk of boredom. It saps vitality and erodes physical and mental health. It is therefore better to risk involvement in reminiscence activities than to do nothing to provide opportunities for stimulation and engagement, even if there is a small likelihood that a small number of individuals might possibly be saddened or upset as a consequence (Bell and Troxel 2004 and 2008).

Reminiscence workers, like oral historians, face the dilemma of whether it is ethical to talk with people for the purpose of recording their recollections, then, once done, abandoning them. There is no simple answer to this dilemma as Yow (2005) and the Oral History Society's guidelines make clear. The guiding principle is founded on the idea of contract. It is better to be open, honest and explicit from the beginning about the purpose of any contract, the nature and likely duration of the relationship, and the nature of the hoped-for outcomes. Most people can accept time limits and time-limited relationships, painful as their ending may be. What no one should be asked to accept is being misled, used and then discarded.

In all such work, the process of engagement needs to be conducted ethically. So too does the production of any tangible outcomes that may also implicate other people who feature in the stories recounted and who may be quite ignorant of what is said about them or unable to defend themselves. Reminiscence workers need to be aware of and to take responsibility for the ethical ramifications of their reminiscence work and to try in every possible way to achieve informed consent – or sometimes in special circumstances assent – on the part of all participants. This consent needs to include an agreement about any tangible outcome, how it will be used, where it will be kept and who may have access to it. Written consent is preferable to verbal consent and the Appendix contains an example.

Conclusion

Many different ways of undertaking reminiscence with individuals and couples have been described including simple reminiscence, structured life review, the combined individual and group method of guided autobiographical writing and life story work. Advances in information and computer technology have greatly increased the scope and ease of producing attractive tangible records in a number of different formats and increasingly people are taking advantage of these new possibilities to create tangible records for their own, their families' and their communities' benefit.

Key points

- Many individuals, couples and families are enriched by the process of making a tangible life record and by the record itself; the processes involved are more important than the tangible outcome or product.

- Various forms of autobiographical, life review and life story work serve as present satisfying activities that create longer-term legacies while also being tools or vehicles through which communication can be improved, relationships enriched and well-being promoted.

- The record can be presented in various formats depending on the objectives to be served, and the interests, energy, expertise and resources available in making it.

- Information and communication technology has much to contribute to accessing, preserving, presenting and archiving life story information.

- The 'product' belongs to the person; access and ownership must be negotiated and respected.

- Signed consent forms are strongly recommended.

- The worker must behave ethically concerning the means and ends, the process and the product.

Application exercises

1. Write down five key words that relate to this chapter. Now write down why these words are important to reminiscence work with individuals, couples or families.

2. What more do you need to learn about or follow up as a result of having read this chapter?

3. Assist someone in making a tangible record of his or her own life story and reflect on what informed the approach used and what benefits accrued for the person, their family and yourself.

Further reading

Bell, V. and Troxel, D. (2008) *The Best Friend's Approach to Alzheimer's Care*. Vol. 11. Baltimore: Health Professions Press.

Birren, J.E. and Deutchman, D. (2005) 'Guided Autobiography Groups.' In B.K. Haight and F. Gibson (eds) *Burnside's Working with Older People: Group Process and Techniques*. Boston: Jones and Bartlett.

Haight, B.K. and Haight, B.S. (2007) *The Handbook of Structured Life Review*. Baltimore: Health Professions Press.

Sherman, J. (2008a) *Computing for Beginners*. London: AgeUK.

Sherman, J. (2008b) *Everyday Computing*. London: AgeUK.

Chapter 8

Reminiscence and Oral History in Community Development

Learning outcomes

After studying this chapter you should be able to:

- explain the use of reminiscence and oral history as tools for promoting community development, understanding community conflict, and promoting social inclusion and mutual understanding
- understand how to apply reminiscence skills to encourage life-long learning and community cohesion and lessen suspicion between groups
- identify the actions required to implement reminiscence projects in community contexts
- appreciate the values that should inform community development, and community and adult education.

Wider community applications of reminiscence and oral history

So far reminiscence work with individuals, couples and small groups for purposes that mostly benefit each individual involved has been considered. This chapter is concerned with adapting and expanding this knowledge so as to benefit a larger number of people. Private troubles or personal problems are re-defined as public issues when a group of people realise that they, and probably other people, share common concerns or face shared issues that need to be addressed in a more public way. The Community Development Foundation considers the purpose of community development as helping groups take action together about matters concerned with the public good, and to assist groups to influence the decisions that affect their lives. (See www.cdf.org.uk.)

Some community development projects use reminiscence and oral history as part of raising community awareness of problems and as means for appreciating the antecedents of social needs and issues, strengthening relationships, developing social cohesion and mobilising resources. It is therefore helpful to appreciate which aspects of reminiscence and oral history are common to both approaches and which are different. Major similarities and differences are summarised in Table 8.1.

Table 8.1: Comparisons between oral history and reminiscence	
Oral history	**Reminiscence**
Intended to preserve and transmit knowledge	Intended to benefit the individual
Major emphasis on outcome product	Major emphasis on relationships and process Secondary interest sometimes on a product
Uses semi-structured interview with prepared questions on a defined topic	Is interactive, less structured, less interrogative, more flexibly responsive and open-ended
Done by history students and oral historians	Done by many different health and social care professionals, oral historians, reminiscence workers, community artists, community development staff, families and volunteers
Usually done with individuals although sometimes in small groups	Usually done in small groups and also with individuals and couples
Ownership of the product usually passes to the interviewer	Ownership is open to negotiation
Power is vested in the interviewer	Power is vested in the participants
Interviewer sets the agenda and directs the interview or group session	Facilitator negotiates a mutually agreed agenda or programme
Legitimises the telling of personal stories and seeks to connect these with documented history or other oral accounts	Celebrates personal stories and is usually less concerned to locate individual accounts within documented public history

Table 8.1 *cont.*	
Awareness of ethical issues governing ends and means	Awareness of ethical issues governing ends and means
Uses various oral and documentary accounts to check veracity and historical accuracy of accounts	Less concerned with truth telling and historical accuracy – more concerned with understanding what the story means to its teller
Always uses audio or video recording and note taking during an interview	Does not always make an audio, video or written record although will usually make some notes, often after a meeting
Seldom uses multi-sensory prompts	Frequently uses multi-sensory prompts
Interviews are frequently done in people's own homes, schools, museums or libraries	Located in many different domestic and community venues including health and social care facilities

Source: Adapted from Bornat (2006) and Gibson (2004).

Community development refers to a process that seeks to encourage social justice, citizenship, participation, empowerment, advocacy, self-help and collective action primarily, but not always, by impoverished, marginalised or socially disadvantaged groups. It seeks to develop knowledge and skills, to build capacity and, by promoting networking and cooperative action, to assist groups and communities to realise their potential or to meet agreed identified needs. It challenges prejudice, racism, sectarianism and unequal distribution of power and access to resources. Communities are encouraged to identify and to tackle problems that are recognised as important at a local neighbourhood level, and to build partnerships with statutory, voluntary and not for profit agencies, and sometimes local business interests, in order to acquire the skills and resources needed to overcome them.

The groups involved in such work are connected because of where they live and the needs of their local neighbourhood or larger community. Sometimes they consist of people who share common characteristics such as ethnicity or disability or a common interest or special need, although the people involved may not live in close proximity to each other. This sort of grouping is known as a community of interest rather than a locality-based or geographically-based group. By working together, groups defined either by locality or interest seek to benefit more people than themselves, their families or those with whom they live in housing, health or care facilities.

This does not exclude benefit for group members and others with whom they are personally connected but the objective is to benefit or improve conditions and quality of life for others as well who may not be directly involved in the change process.

Much of the earlier material concerning reminiscence work is relevant to its use in community development contexts but some objectives and the nature of the contract are likely to be different. Community development is a set of activities or actions that assists individuals, groups and communities to achieve positive social change for the public benefit. It challenges suspicion of difference, works to broaden opportunities for public participation, and seeks to promote understanding between diverse people in order to promote the common good. It challenges racism, poverty, marginalisation and divisiveness and promotes social inclusion and responsible citizenship. It does not deny differences but rather seeks to celebrate, value and share both common and separate characteristics as a means of bringing about social cohesion, change and development.

We too easily feel threatened by differences of age, class, culture, education, income, language, race, religion, sexual orientation, upbringing and values. Yet we do not need to be captives of our heritage and history. If we are to live peaceably in a threatened and threatening world, understanding of difference and generosity towards others of divergent backgrounds is essential at community, national and international levels.

Learning from history

Oral history and reminiscence can make a considerable contribution towards enhancing community understanding and achieving the social inclusion of disparate groups. By assisting individuals to discover and value their own history and personal identity it becomes more possible for them to reach out to others. Through sharing stories together, different and common experiences emerge. This can become the catalyst for shared effort in identifying problems and then solving problems – essential processes for building cohesive communities. Reminiscence with an oral history emphasis can never be the sole means used in community development. It can, however, make a very worthwhile contribution both in terms of understanding local neighbourhoods and communities, the backgrounds of the persons involved and the problems requiring attention, and building community capacity in order to address them.

If we can understand the past we may better understand the present and be more able to plan for the future. Making comparisons between the past and the present seems to be a natural response when we experience stress in the present, regardless of age or type of threat. This stress stimulates problem solving. If anxiety becomes too great when faced with overwhelming stress, individuals and groups may need assistance in order to trigger recall, to remember past coping and to be able to make and to learn from past and present comparisons. If individuals and groups fail to learn from the past, they are likely to experience the present as threatening, be fearful of the future and liable to repeat the mistakes of the past.

Characteristics of community-based reminiscence workers

Reminiscence and oral history projects located in community contexts seek to encourage exploration of the past, including dominant attitudes, values and behaviour. They facilitate change or modification through exploring personal, group and communal folk memories that separate and alienate people from one another. Doing history with community groups requires workers to be:

- secure in their own identity – aware of the impact of their own history and unthreatened by difference
- confident in handling conflict
- willing to hold people to the exploration of memories, no matter how painful
- able to think critically and be open to developing new perspectives
- sufficiently secure to question informants and the partisan views they may be expressing
- willing to question the role and relevance of history, oral history and reminiscence work
- confident in challenging conventional prevailing accounts of history
- able to ensure that conflicting accounts and alternative interpretations of history are heard
- skilled in raising issues about representation and the possible impact of the stories on others
- persistent in assisting participants to understand that there is more than one version of a story, even if one version predominates

- willing to encourage people to examine their own views of history, especially if they come to hold a view that diverges from the dominant one

- patient in negotiating how material will be represented and how discordant voices can also be heard and accommodated.

Life-long learning, reminiscence and oral history

Much adult education or life-long learning which sometimes is known as community education or informal education has always been closely allied to the provision of second chance education and training that is designed to achieve various purposes ranging from second chance opportunities for disadvantaged learners, recreation, skill acquisition and skill updating, and achieving greater community coherence and inclusion. Many programmes are closely allied with community development and commonly utilise oral and local history as part of their curriculum. Often the line between oral history and reminiscence in community-based adult learning is blurred and which term is preferred depends more on the affiliation and identity of the provider organisation than on the focus or content of study. Housden (2007) describes many different ways in which reminiscence and oral history have been embedded in educational activities and projects for adult learners including community organisations, public libraries, museums, day centres and care homes. The Heritage Lottery Fund and the Big Lottery have supported innumerable oral history projects and associated publications and exhibitions, many using explicit reminiscence group work approaches, throughout the UK. Many accounts of such projects have been published over the years in *Oral History,* the journal of the Oral History Society (see www.ohs.org.uk). In years to come, as efforts to control global warming increase in urgency, older people's accounts of life in earlier, less affluent, less profligate times are likely to become valuable sources of information and guidance.

Project management

Most community-based reminiscence and oral history work is organised on a project basis. In achieving successful outcomes, efficient project management, regardless of the size or duration of a project, is important, in addition to being knowledgeable about reminiscence and oral history. There is no such thing as a standard plan or magic formula which guarantees success of a project although a framework or template can assist in keeping a project on course. It is increasingly common in large projects to use standardised formats, or computer software such as Microsoft Project which comes as a standard part of MS Office, to guide a project. Even if experienced in project development and management a template or framework can be helpful. The key stages and processes involved are:

- project initiation
- project plan
- facilitate and coordinate the implementation and execution
- monitor and review
- integrate changes
- close project.

Planning needs to include arrangements for securing, spending and accounting for resources used, arrangements for record keeping and reporting agreed and a realistic timetable established. Enthusiastic project initiators should think carefully about the resources needed as these are too frequently underestimated. They also need to identify any potential financial or other risks which might be incurred and to formulate an exigency plan. By finally evaluating a project its quality and costs can be assessed, as well as benefits for participants, skills gained, mistakes identified, lessons learned, tools and techniques refined and desirable future changes identified.

The most frequent reasons underlying project failure are:

- inadequate preparation and planning
- erroneous or insufficient identification of need and project objectives
- lack of an explicit agreement or 'contract' with sponsors, funders and participants
- lack of clarity about roles and responsibilities of facilitators and other helpers
- inaccurate budget forecasting and accountability
- lack of confidence and skill in evaluating positive and negative features
- insufficient feedback to participants and resource providers on completion.

This is particularly relevant to reminiscence and oral history work within a community development framework. Building effective relationships with individuals and partnerships with community groups and statutory, voluntary and private organisations are essential skills (Carnwell and Buchanan 2004). This requires getting to know the community, its formal and informal organisations and their leaders, the economic, social and health needs of the area existing resources and how they are distributed. Involving other agencies in partnership projects requires a basic knowledge of key people and relevant organisations. A starter list for a reminiscence network should include community groups, health, social care, arts, faith and cultural organisations, libraries, museums, schools and colleges, and local business leaders, politicians and municipal officials.

Initially it is helpful to think in broad terms and then systematically refine the search for key people from other organisations in terms of what social problem needs to be addressed or what objectives need to be achieved. Think of a series of concentric circles as in Figure 8.1 – the inner one representing a group of people or a neighbourhood with a problem that requires attention. In seeking to initiate any particular project, already established networks are likely to be considered first but it is also helpful to think afresh and at the project initiation stage to identify how other service systems might possibly be involved. When planning a group or project begin to identify in ever widening circles relevant resource organisations and relevant people within them who may be interested in working in partnership.

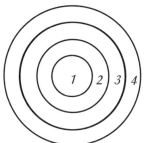

Key
1. Group with interest, issue or problem for work
2. Local neighbourhood resources
3. Regional resource organisations
4. National resource organisations

Figure 8.1: Identifying and locating community resources

Enhancing practice through developing partnerships

Many professionals find that one of the most attractive aspects of reminiscence group work is its wide appeal to members of many different professions and occupations. It provides wonderfully rich opportunities for mixing with, learning from and being challenged by people whose training and work experience may be substantially different. Initially this may be disconcerting, less comfortable and more complex than choosing to work with familiar people of similar background. Multi-disciplinary and inter-agency collaboration can be very fruitful although learning to work cooperatively and constructively across organisational boundaries usually requires considerable effort. Relationships grow when purposeful work is shared with mutually respectful and responsible partners. This does not mean that everyone is equal in terms of knowledge, skills, experience or responsibilities. It does mean, however, that there is clarity and explicit understanding about the contribution expected from each person in the team, and the resources they can bring, be they a professional or a volunteer, a senior practitioner or a new worker.

A mixture of people from various backgrounds and agencies usually proves fruitful and releases creative, imaginative ideas and novel ways of doing reminiscence. Librarians, museum staff, health and social care practitioners and community workers frequently pool resources and collaborate productively. Housing staff, teachers and community arts workers contribute immensely to the success of many reminiscence and oral history projects. Volunteers of all ages are especially valuable. They tend to bring a reassurance to participants who may be inherently suspicious of 'professionals' or 'outsiders'. Volunteers must be given pivotal responsibilities and not left to feel undervalued – just invited along to make the tea or provide the transport – as important as these tasks are.

Oral history and reminiscence have been used in many different countries and for exploring and clarifying many different types of communal problems or issues. Some examples include efforts designed to challenge sectarianism and foster cross-community relations and mutual understanding in Northern Ireland, establishing land rights by Aboriginal Australians, integrating successive waves of immigrant groups in New York, seeking to reconcile past wrongs in post apartheid South Africa, and reducing energy demands by learning from earlier simpler lifestyles (Gibson 2004).

Conclusion

Reminiscence and oral history, although developing from different academic and professional traditions, nevertheless share many common values, objectives and methods. Differences in approach, objectives, structure, formats for gathering, recording and interpreting data and sometimes in the people and contexts involved have been identified. Both are used extensively in community development and life-long learning projects that encourage people to reflect upon their personal and communal memories in efforts to understand, reconstruct and reconcile contested and uncontested representations of history. The approaches are used as pathways for informing members of community partnerships and networks in their efforts to understand and overcome present problems and meet the identified needs of local groups and communities.

Key points

- Reminiscence and oral history and life-long learning have overlapping objectives, methods and values.
- Communities, whether constituted by shared geography or commitment to seeking improvements or change concerning common issues or shared needs, use reminiscence and oral history as vehicles for understanding past experience and engaging in problem solving in the present.
- Project management and networking skills are needed to engage in effective work within communities.
- Working in cooperative community-wide partnerships can be more effective than working in isolation.

Application exercises

1. Identify a concern or problem raised by an individual, family, small group or organisation that may have similar implications for other people. Consider what relevance oral history or reminiscence may have in achieving greater understanding of the problem and efforts to seek a solution.

2. Identify any other accessible resource organisations and key people whose help might be enlisted in undertaking an oral history or reminiscence project.

3. List the possible advantages and disadvantages of seeking and obtaining their involvement as partners in a reminiscence project designed to achieve an identified community objective.

Further reading

Harris, V. (2006) *Practice and Principles in Community Development Work: Resource Pack 10*. Sheffield: Confederation for Community Development Learning.

Housden., S. (2007) *Reminiscence and Lifelong Learning*. Leicester: NIACE.

Popple, K. and Quinney, A. (2006) 'Community development in the 21st century.' *British Journal of Social Work 36*, 2, 333–340.

Thompson, P. (2005) *The Voice of the Past*. Oxford: Oxford University Press.

Chapter 9

Reminiscence with People from Minority Ethnic Groups

Learning outcomes

After studying this chapter you should be able to:

- list reasons why reminiscence with members of minority ethnic groups is valuable
- understand why it is important to be aware of cultural differences towards ageing, death and dying
- understand the challenges faced by people who are growing old in a second homeland
- explain the importance of bearing witness to personal, family and group experiences
- identify the advantages and complexities of co-working in groups with a membership drawn from different ethnic backgrounds.

Acquiring background knowledge

To be an effective reminiscence worker with people from different ethnic groups it is important to learn about their history, religion, values, beliefs, customs and traditions. Broad general knowledge can only provide a background as there are innumerable differences both within and between ethnic groups. Before starting any group it is important to be as well informed as possible about the likely origins and possible experiences of the people involved (see Chapters 5 and 6). But however much is learned, it is essential to remember that this information may not apply to the actual individuals in a particular reminiscence group or project. Some knowledge of twentieth century

British colonial history, and recent and current immigration and asylum policies, will assist understanding why people from varied countries and backgrounds live in the United Kingdom and what significance this holds for them. Getting to know individual people from different backgrounds will help prevent stereotyping. It will help you learn to appreciate each person as a unique individual, not just as a member of an ethnic group to which are ascribed general characteristics. It should be appreciated that the National Health Service, local authority social services departments and many other British organisations would fail to function effectively if not staffed by people from other countries.

In all successful reminiscence work, respect for people, regardless of age, race, culture, religion, politics, gender and sexual orientation, is essential. Discriminatory attitudes and behaviour are unacceptable, and sensitive anti-discriminatory practice will be essential should racism, or any other form of discrimination, surface in a reminiscence group.

Benefits from ethnic elders sharing their recollections

There are many reasons for encouraging ethnic elders to share their recollections. Schweitzer (1998a) suggests these include:

- countering social isolation by developing two-way relationships and friendships
- providing tools for building community identity
- helping to develop memorabilia collections that are relevant to minority and majority communities
- keeping a culture alive and vibrant by passing on learning, guidance and wisdom
- giving a sense of self-worth and cultural identity for generations to come, for example through passing on cultural traditions such as story telling
- making connections across cultural, spiritual, generational and linguistic barriers
- hearing the voices of older minority people so that they can claim and reclaim their own histories
- overcoming racist myths and stereotypes

- assisting incomers to value themselves and to be respected by others
- helping to make services more responsive to people's varied needs.

Cultural differences towards ageing, death and dying

The experience of death is universal. The experience of how it is responded to varies in innumerable ways depending upon culture, religion, custom and conviction, and informed by memory and re-enacted in experience.

Being invited to tell one's story is likely to evoke different responses in people from different ethnic backgrounds. For some it may be a natural thing to do, for others it may seem a strange or peculiar invitation. There may also be class, caste, gender and educational differences, so do not expect everyone to respond in the same way just because they belong to the same minority ethnic group. Be prepared to appreciate minority individual and group differences.

If people share a common heritage, common origins, language and values, group work is likely to be more spontaneous than it might otherwise be in a more heterogeneous group. Many people with similar ethnic backgrounds will probably enjoy reminiscing with each other immensely but reminiscence work in a group of people from different ethnic backgrounds is possible and often very desirable.

Reminiscence work as outlined in this book, with its emphasis on personal life history, albeit shared with others, however, may seem strangely western and therefore alien or irrelevant to older people from some other cultural traditions. Not for everyone does the life lived give meaning to old age. Respect for elders and valuing the wisdom they have attained will be very important in some societies, but not in all. Consider carefully the culture and traditions of the people likely to be involved, and adapt the objectives, style and content of the intended reminiscence work accordingly. For example, white British and Asian elders may approach old age and death differently; they may not view life satisfaction in the same way nor share the same ideas about the meaning of their own lives or the meaning of life in general. Do not expect everyone to believe or accept dominant western ideas. Many westerners, for example, believe that there is one and only one life while followers of some other world religions believe there are many previous and future lives.

There are also varied views about how much people as they age should remain busily absorbed in everyday life. Contemplation rather than active engagement in late life is preferred in some cultures where withdrawal and seclusion rather than engagement and sociability are the norm. Disengagement rather than activity may be more desired.

In some eastern religions a sense of personal fulfilment and absence of fear about the future, especially fear of death, is more publicly expressed, and religion is less private and personal than in the west. Older people from non-Christian backgrounds may find the western emphasis on personal recollection and individual life history very odd and very self-centred. They may have a greater sense of community, of family, of being connected to others, and reminiscence work needs to be sensitive to these different traditions.

Growing old in a second homeland

The life story connects each person to place and culture. If these connections have been disrupted for whatever reason, perhaps because of war, abuse, escape, becoming a refugee, migration, or separation from home or family, it is particularly important to help people reconnect with their past and to be encouraged to remember significant relationships and once familiar places.

Most people who experience loss of significant places, even when freely chosen for positive rather than negative reasons, feel a kind of grief, or what Read (1996) calls 'bereavement of place'. Workers' own awareness of lost places, near or far, of being 'strangers' in unfamiliar surroundings or circumstances, of paths not taken, or opportunities lost, may help them to appreciate, in some small way, the sense of loss, anxiety and dislocation experienced by others.

Growing old in a second homeland or growing old as a member of a minority ethnic group, even if born in Britain, may mean being disadvantaged and discriminated against in many different ways. Generally, people from all backgrounds who are healthy, well housed, have a close confidant and are economically secure do best in later life. Many immigrants and asylum seekers may experience poor health and poor housing and have had a long history of poorly paid employment or unemployment which results in an inadequate and insecure old age. Many do not manage to get adequate help from public services so in late life feel unsupported and vulnerable. Having lost a homeland, they may not have gained a secure, respected place in their adopted country.

Group reminiscence for people from ethnic minorities may therefore be an important way of reconnecting them with their own communities and reaffirming their own historical and cultural roots. If managed sensitively, reminiscence work may help to convey a sense of respect, warmth and genuine interest in cultural diversity. It can help confirm both common and different characteristics and help people to value their life experience and cultural heritage. If workers are insensitive or treat people in ways experienced as or perceived to be disrespectful, or even racist, the older person from a different culture will feel hurt, alienated and demeaned.

Some care workers find it hard to empathise with an older person if past relationships with older people have been sparse or negative. This problem will be exacerbated if a lack of knowledge about immigration or first-hand acquaintance with immigrants is added. Alternatively, a worker may belong to a minority ethnic group, even if born in Britain. Whatever a person's age, ethnic origin and life experience may be, everyone needs to be open to learning about 'difference' and to appreciate how we feel and behave towards people who are 'different' from ourselves.

> We differ from one another in race, in national origin, in ethnicity, in gender, in sexual orientation, in beliefs, in political loyalties, in abilities, in personal histories, and in many other ways. These differences must be acknowledged and respected. The most profound and enduring truth is what we have in common, and what we have in common is our humanity. (Lynn 2001, p.22)

Many immigrants, refugees and asylum seekers regard their new country with mixed feelings. Some may be proud and well satisfied with their achievements. For some who may have experienced economic hardship, ill health, racism and loneliness, living in Britain may have been an unhappy, unrewarding, lonely experience, now made worse by lack of adequate care in old age.

Some 'newcomers' may feel failures in their new land. They may experience a deep, probably unattainable, nostalgic, longing to return to their homeland. Many realise the place they have left will no longer be the same, even if they could afford to return. Difficulties overcome, personal fulfilment and family success should be applauded. Reminiscence work uncovers pain but also provides many openings for affirmation, validation, encouragement and recognition of courage and achievement.

Immigration is not inevitably and universally perceived in terms of loss. Even in the face of much hardship endured, it will seldom be seen as totally negative. More often, leaving home, migrating, settling and growing old in a foreign land is spoken of with mixed or ambivalent feelings. These experiences are usually reported as a mixture of pain and pleasure, loss and gain, relinquishment, courageous new beginnings and small triumphs; any perceived ambivalence expressed in words or gestures needs to be accepted and openly acknowledged and achievements validated.

Learning from minority ethnic elders
Be finely tuned to the older person in the here and now; to understand what their present, as well as past, concerns are and be willing to share that experience, at the pace and in the ways in which the person wishes to recount it.

Take the time to learn about different ethnic groups as well as to understand about the personal life experience of any particular individual. One effective way of gaining this knowledge is to listen attentively to older people from minority ethnic communities talking about their own homelands. Ask them questions; try to appreciate what life used to be like for them and in what ways it has changed.

Much of the fine detail of their stories will be affected by each individual's present circumstances and how receptive he or she perceives the audience to be. When reminiscing careful selection of triggers will be necessary so that the homeland as well as the new land is represented.

Families, community groups, churches, synagogues, mosques and temples, local radio stations, especially those serving ethnic groups, embassies, consulates, museums and libraries may be able to assist in locating culturally relevant background materials and multi-sensory triggers.

The same guidelines about group membership, good communication and building relationships already mentioned in earlier chapters apply to work with members drawn from a single ethnic group or from various ethnic groups. If the leaders of a multi-ethnic group share the same background as some of the members, difficulties of communication and language will obviously be lessened. If the facilitator is a 'stranger', this is an opportunity for the older people to become the teachers in a very important sense.

There is likely to be only a small number of people from any particular minority ethnic group in most day centres, care homes and hospitals. Nevertheless, even if small in number, their different needs concerning language, information, food, hygiene, hair care, religious observance, health care, death and mourning customs and rituals need sensitive attention. Henley and Schott's (2004) *Culture, Religion and Patient Care in a Multi-ethnic Society* provides a wealth of relevant information.

Religious festivals such as Eid ul-Fitr and Eid al-Adha (Muslim), Diwali and Holi (Hindu) and Passover and Hanukkah (Jewish) can provide opportunities for reminiscence about past celebrations in distant places as well as being opportunities for valuing a person's special identity and extending understanding. Celebrations involving music, song, dance, storytelling, readings, recitals, films and food could focus on events like Caribbean independence days, Chinese New Year, St Andrew's Day, St David's Day, St Patrick's Day and many other special occasions.

Achieving cultural continuity by means of teaching and passing on traditions to inform and influence the next generation is very important in many reminiscence projects with people from minority ethnic groups. Reminiscence can also assist with linking the past with the present, in problem solving, relationship building and coming to terms with life as it has turned out. Reminiscence as problem solving may be especially relevant to older people who live in care homes or attend day centres that are not finely tuned to individuals' cultural, dietary and religious needs, preferences and interests. Reminiscence can become a constructive means for recognising and honouring different traditions and for influencing carers to enable them to respond more appropriately to the diverse needs and wishes of their residents or service users.

The day centre coordinator for the League of Jewish Women described how:

Often past lives were talked about for the first time in our reminiscence group. Non-Jewish staff could join in and make comparisons with their own past and tell of their own religious traditions. Probably the most important spin-off was the opportunity it gave to care staff and social workers to understand more about the different world their residents and clients had come from.

Reminiscence as life review may be too painful for some, but helpful for those who can bear to speak about their past experience and its joys and disappointments. They may have endured enormous loss and suffering and it may take immigrants or refugees longer to trust themselves to talk about their deepest concerns. Some may not wish to share their life review, for them a private solitary process, particularly if they have had a hard struggle to come to terms with life's pain. Some may feel caught in a struggle to live life in two places, of wanting desperately to hang on to their old traditions while needing to accommodate their present changed circumstances (Blackwell 2005). It may be helpful to refer back to Chapter 4 on different styles and Chapter 7 on methods of reminiscing as autobiographical writing, structured and unstructured life review and life story work may suit some people better than group reminiscence.

The importance of bearing witness

Many immigrants and refugees have an overwhelming urge to 'bear witness'. For some, their pain has been so terrible, their loss so great, that it takes them many years to be able to speak about the enormity of their suffering. This has been seen most frequently, but not only, with Jewish survivors of the Nazi Holocaust and war veterans from many countries. With continued wars, terrorism, famine, persecution, genocide, population displacement, abuse, torture and man-made and natural disasters of many kinds in many parts of the world, similar reactions from increasing numbers of people to extreme trauma can be anticipated in the years ahead.

Some survivors find that no amount of telling can diminish their suffering, while others are quite unable to break their silence and to speak of the unspeakable. 'Why was I spared?' and 'How could it happen?' may become recurring preoccupations in later life when there is more time for looking back and for introspection. Reminiscence in intergenerational family groups is particularly relevant although often very complex. Putting the record straight, telling it as it was by at last breaking the silence, is one way of honouring the dead, validating the experience, and justifying the survival of the witness. Such work is very demanding; it requires great skill and workers undertaking it require competent supportive supervision.

Some writers have suggested that people who have endured terrible suffering or extreme trauma are sometimes unable to speak about it to their children but eventually, long after the event, are able to speak to their grandchildren. Hunt *et al.* (1997) give many case examples of people who in earlier life experienced various kinds of trauma, which emerged only in late life or, for some, re-emerged in late life when they were overtaken by dementia.

Always remember that some people manage to survive in the present only by forgetting the past – for them remembering is to be avoided. Some descendants of survivors distance themselves from the stories of their elders – they cannot bear to hear because they do not wish to carry the burdens of history; for them, living in the present is more important. There is still much to learn about the timing and the context in which traumatic life stories come to be told. Bearing witness, advising others and at last feeling that the time has come to break the silence was demonstrated by Harry Patch, the last WWI veteran who died aged 111 on 5 August 2009. When interviewed on BBC Radio 4 at 4.00pm on 25 December 2005 he said: 'I went for 80 years and I never spoke of the World War – not even to my wife.' People's timing must be respected but it is, however, absolutely essential that, when the time to speak comes, there are skilled and sensitive listeners willing to hear the stories people now feel compelled to tell (Wave 2010).

Co-working and trans-cultural facilitation

White reminiscence workers facilitating minority ethnic or mixed race groups may unknowingly be perceived as dominating, condescending or oppressive, so they must take particular care to be well informed about the backgrounds of group members. They need to be aware of their own attitudes and prejudices, and to be sensitive and open to new learning. One care worker said:

> We need to be aware of our own feelings. We need to be honest about how we feel about older people generally and race in particular if we are to ease some of the hurt.

Any co-working relationship is complex, as has already been explained in Chapter 5. If facilitators differ from each other in ethnic background the implications require careful exploration at the planning stage. What mix of age, class and gender is likely to be feasible and acceptable? Should the group and its leaders be all black or Asian, all white or black and white? Some groupworkers, both black and white, question whether black/white co-working is ever possible or acceptable. It is important to know where facilitators stand on such issues so they are not caught unawares when becoming involved in reminiscence group work. Mistry and Brown (1991) suggest that black/white co-worker pairing is usually desirable where the group is racially mixed and there are many potential benefits associated with joint working.

Co-working in all reminiscence groups requires explicit consideration of the following concerns:

- Are potential facilitators willing and able to model co-facilitation?
- Have they discussed general ground rules?
- How many workers are proposed; should it be one, two or more?
- Is a black/white pair appropriate?
- Can facilitators work comfortably with each other?
- Are they likely to agree on purpose, principles and practice?
- Can they talk openly about the race dimension of the partnership?
- Have they talked about issues of authority between themselves and within the group?
- Have they agreed how to handle racism if it becomes an issue within the group?
- Have they agreed how differences in background, aptitudes, skill, experience and ability are to be managed between the co-workers?
- Have they planned to rotate and share tasks so that the white worker will not automatically be cast as the leader in the eyes of the members?
- Is each likely to be able to offer and accept honest feedback on performance?
- Are arrangements about supervision and consultation agreed?

Overcoming barriers to effective work

The experience of all immigrants will not be the same, even though they all share the common elements of leaving, journeying, arriving, settling and the feeling of never completely belonging. To be old in Britain and to be Irish, Polish, Chinese, Asian, African, Somali or Caribbean will not be the same experience. Do not assume that reminiscing with one minority group will be any easier than reminiscing with any other, just because the facilitator shares a common first language. Shared language obviously helps but many other subtle factors are also important. Again Henley and Schott (2004) give detailed information about cultural, linguistic, religious and other ethnic differences as well as guidance about working with interpreters. They stress the need to develop sensitivity to personal biases, prejudices and language limitations.

Reminiscence groups that touch on the harsh realities of discrimination may be hard for white facilitators and members to cope with because their own racial attitudes and national identity will be challenged. Accounts of prejudice, discrimination and racism at work or school, abuse, violence, being refused accommodation and denied employment and educational opportunities or care which others take for granted are liable to arouse guilt, defensiveness or denial. Both tellers and hearers will be touched and challenged in many different ways. Effective group work demands accepting that feelings, no matter how painful and threatening, are openly talked about and honestly acknowledged.

Take particular care to overcome any language or other communication barriers so that anyone who wishes to participate is not excluded from reminiscence work. Invitations and notices may need to be written in various languages depending on who is to be invited. Besides English, the most common languages and dialects spoken in the UK are probably Bengali, Cantonese, Gujarati, Hindi, Kutchi, Mandarin, Patois, Polish, Punjabi, Sylheti and Urdu but there may be many others including various European languages.

Consider using interpreters. When looking for assistance with interpretation, begin near at hand. Are there work colleagues who speak the required language who could be asked to help? If not, look elsewhere. Some local authorities and health trusts provide interpreter services. Many social services fieldwork teams employ social workers from varied ethnic backgrounds. Local community groups and language agencies may be pleased to become involved as volunteers. Schools and faith groups may be delighted to volunteer assistance in order to create opportunities for community service or intergenerational projects which are dealt with more fully in Chapter 10.

Conclusion

The courage, resilience and strength of people, especially those from minority ethnic groups, need to be recognised and celebrated. Reminiscence as witnessing, teaching, problem solving, identity preservation and for improving self-esteem can greatly contribute to well-being. It can be a bridge to connect the person to his or her culture, both past and present. People whose lives have been disrupted by geographic dispersal, emigration and separation from home and family may find group reminiscence or individual life review particularly helpful. Some of their earlier experience of pain and loss may be mirrored in late life – and possibly reactivated for some – by the pain of other life events such as divorce, bereavement, ill health, disability or admission to care. Having the opportunity to reconnect via reminiscence and recall to important past events, significant relationships and special places may make the present more agreeable or at least more tolerable.

Ethnically sensitive reminiscence work will not solve all the problems associated with inequality, racism and social exclusion. It is, however, a way of challenging discrimination, extending mutual understanding and establishing warm, respectful, caring relationships. This will not happen automatically or effortlessly, but only as we confront our own prejudices and are open to learning from people whose race, beliefs, language, religion, culture and life experience differ from our own. Small reminiscence groups and individual life story work offer a sympathetic climate in which this process might begin.

Key points

- Be alert to the possibility of imposing majority cultural values on others.
- Develop understanding about what it is like to grow old in a second homeland through reading, sensitive questioning and careful listening.

- Ethnically sensitive reminiscence work can help to inform about differences of religion, ethnicity, age, gender, class and status.
- Cross-cultural groups can share common life experiences if not a shared cultural inheritance.
- Intergenerational and cross-cultural work can be rewarding for people of all ages.
- Co-leadership that reflects the ethnicity of the participants is commended but requires careful preparation and honest implementation.

Application exercises

1. Find an older person whose ethnic origin differs from your own. Ask if he or she will teach you about the important aspects of his or her culture, especially attitudes and practices concerned with family life, age and ageing, death and dying.

2. Begin to develop a co-working relationship with a colleague whose ethnic background differs from your own. Try reading and then discussing this chapter together before commencing joint reminiscence work.

3. Plan to do some reminiscence, life review or life story work with an older person(s) from a minority ethnic group. Prepare a list of possible relevant multi-sensory triggers which are age, gender, geographically and culturally appropriate and identify where you might locate them.

Further reading

Henley, A. and Schott, J. (2004) *Culture, Religion and Patient Care in a Multi-ethnic Society: A Handbook for Professionals*. London: Age Concern.

Mistry, T. and Brown, A. (eds) (1996) *Race and Groupwork*. London: Whiting and Birch.

O'Hagan, K. (2001) *Cultural Competence in the Caring Professions*. London: Jessica Kingsley Publishers.

Schweitzer, P. (ed.) (1998) *The Journey of a Lifetime*. London: European Reminiscence Network.

Chapter 10

Intergenerational Reminiscence Work

Learning outcomes

After studying this chapter you should be able to:

- develop awareness of the significance of informal reminiscence within families
- understand the opportunities and obstacles in doing planned reminiscence work with individuals, pairs or groups of people of different ages
- appreciate that careful preparation for intergenerational reminiscence work is essential
- formulate a tentative plan for an intergenerational reminiscence project so as to be ready to embark on such a project.

The mutual benefits of intergenerational reminiscing

Although intergenerational solidarity is a much vaunted public policy objective it seems that ambivalence, indifference and sometimes outright hostility between different age groups may be a more accurate description of some people's experience. Contact between older and younger people may be driven by duty, obligation and self-interest as much as by familial or neighbourly altruism, affection, concern and friendship. Too many children, lacking close personal ties with an older person, risk adopting and perpetuating the myths and stereotypes about ageing which still persist in present day society. Despite such pessimistic views many older people enjoy close satisfying relations with children and younger adults both inside and outside their families and varied organised intergenerational projects are also slowly growing in numbers and in popularity.

Planned intergenerational projects utilising older people as living resources, models and mentors have much to offer both young and old, individuals, families, neighbourhoods and society. Increasingly, the value of enduring benefits for children and adolescents' life-long emotional development, self-esteem, attachment and confidence gained from informal reminiscing within families is recognised (Bluck and Alea 2008; Quas and Fivush 2009). The value of reminiscence and life story work with adopted and fostered children has already been mentioned in Chapter 7.

Reminiscing within families assists young children to develop a sense of personal identity – who they are. Mothers who engage in detailed or elaborated reminiscing with their children encourage the child's capacity to organise their memories into coherent stories, to appreciate, integrate and evaluate the emotions linked to these memories, and so be better equipped to regulate their future emotions rather than being overwhelmed by them. Such reminiscing provides the basis of longer-term autobiographical memory, the development of a dynamic yet enduring stable sense of self and for sustaining well-being.

Younger and older people who engage in intergenerational work report considerable benefits and satisfaction, once their initial anxieties have been overcome. Children of all ages and students in all kinds of schools, including children with special educational needs, benefit in many different ways from direct involvement in reminiscing with older people. Many projects build partnerships between schools and local health and social care facilities including hospitals, care homes, day centres and community groups. Establishing effective working relationships between staff from educational and health care sectors requires time and meticulous attention. Mutual understanding, respect and affection grow out of shared experience – it seldom exists from the outset of a project.

A great deal of intergenerational work takes place within single-identity minority ethnic communities and is designed primarily for elders to teach younger people about cultural traditions, beliefs and values. Members of the white majority culture also recognise the importance of cross-generational work designed to combat ageism, lessen mutual suspicion, build friendships, stimulate mutual concern, and transmit knowledge, experience and wisdom.

Some projects may be both cross-cultural and intergenerational. The value of intergenerational projects is not limited to preserving and passing on language, heritage, history and culture of people from minority ethnic groups, although the need for doing so may be felt more urgently within these communities as children and grandchildren, born in Britain, are increasingly assimilated. Mixing people of different ages and different ethnic and cultural backgrounds together in reminiscence projects can be a fruitful way of promoting trust between members of different communities because by exchanging lifetime experiences and identifying common aspirations suspicions are lessened.

Teaching and transmitting wisdom is frequently given as the major justification for older people's involvement in intergenerational work but such learning is never one sided and should never be portrayed as such. Younger people may learn from older people but the reverse is also true and younger people have much to teach their elders. The ingrained long-established prejudices of older people, for instance religious sectarianism or racial superiority that all too readily have been transmitted across the generations, are being effectively challenged in some communities by the more generous liberal inclusive attitudes of younger people. Older people may need considerable encouragement before being willing to become involved in intergenerational groups or feel they have done nothing of value that would interest younger people. They may initially find it hard to appreciate the mutual benefits of the two-way learning that occurs. Children and young people may also need to be encouraged to perceive themselves as both learners and teachers and not just as 'being nice to old people'. Even if an intergenerational project has a primary reminiscence focus this may well widen to include other unforeseen outcomes. For example, a project with a local history focus evolved to include older members passing on ballroom dancing skills to teenagers preparing for a school formal and the young people reciprocating by teaching the older people how to text with their mobile phones.

Such mutual benefits can be enjoyed by all age groups from pre-school, primary, secondary and tertiary levels as demonstrated by a project worker:

Reminiscence loan boxes from a local museum became the focus for bringing together 16 members of a senior citizens' club and 23 children from a pre-school playgroup. In three small groups the boxes were unpacked and the seniors talked about chosen items while describing their lives when aged three or four. Prompted by the items, the seniors then acted out games, butter making, apple picking and dressing up which the children then enthusiastically played out with great pleasure and mutual interest. An equally lively subsequent session focused on memories of Christmas past when the children were agog at the idea of Santa filling a stocking only with an apple, orange and a piece of chocolate. 'That really brought me back to life' summed up the general pleasure experienced by the seniors with the play group leader commenting on the concentration, attention and avid interest shown by the children.

Similar mutual benefits are identified in the following quotations from Schweitzer (1993, p.7):

Lilian Burnett, school volunteer:

> You are giving them a little bit of your experience. You can tell them and explain it and they're really hanging on what you're saying, as long as you're telling the truth, that's the main thing. You must tell them the absolute truth.

Bill O'Rourke, school volunteer:

> Memories do matter, if we are not to forget our past, if we are to understand and respect one another, because the old are important and the young have things to learn from them.

Betty Green, a primary school pupil:

> I love the days our friends from the day centre come to school – we all do things together and help each other. They tell us stories and then we usually draw together or we draw and they chat, and we tell them what games we play and sing our favourite songs which they are now learning from us.

Eileen O'Sullivan, school volunteer:

> I find it gives me a lot of confidence when I tell the children my experience. I feel really great. I couldn't do that with grown up people, but with children I come over well and I feel as though I have done something.

Projects vary in objectives, size, duration, complexity and resources required. Some are undertaken within the school day as part of the National Curriculum while others utilise students' leisure time and may occur in a variety of venues including youth clubs, community arts organisations, museums, care homes and people's own homes (Savill 2002). If the work takes place within an educational setting, it conveys to children and to older people that it is valued. If it takes place within a health or social care facility, it will convey messages of frailty and illness, hopefully tempered by resilience and an enduring capacity for having fun. If it takes place within a family it recognises and contributes to family solidarity, affection, regard and care. Intergenerational work takes many different forms and brings social as well as educational benefits. Older people are able to share their knowledge of varied life experience, history, geography and other subjects with younger people who appreciate hearing vivid first-hand accounts of past times. For example:

> At the end of the project's celebration evening in the library I was speaking to one of the children's mothers, who told me how her daughter had gone missing while on a recent visit to a relative in a nursing home. After a brief search the little girl was found in the main hall. 'There she was...holding court with all the elderly residents, taking notes and recording them in the notebook she had brought specifically for the job.' (Quinn 2010 p.22)

Children are intrigued and captivated by hearing first-hand accounts of past times and events. YouTube provides easily accessible material on a vast array of interesting relevant topics to intrigue, stimulate and focus family conversations across the generations as reported by a consultant geriatrician who is now supporting young staff to experiment with using a similar approach with older patients in an acute hospital setting (Collins *et al.* 2010).

The importance of careful preparation for everyone involved

Careful preparation of everyone involved is not a dispensable 'extra'. Initial separate preparation of both older and younger people is critical for success. Only when each group has faced their anxiety and shared their reservations will they be ready to meet each other. Preliminary exercises that explore stereotypes usually assist each group to develop trust and willingness to move into joint meetings.

In preparing the older informants for a first meeting – for example, a school visit, a preliminary reminiscence session on the same theme as the intended school topic – we help them to realise they have much to tell. By talking about their own stories and listening to the stories of their peers, further memories will surface so that the eventual exchanges in school are likely to be much more detailed. Encourage the older people to visualise the children they will be meeting, to practise adapting the presentation of their stories accordingly and to respond to questions in expansive rather than limited ways. The older informants need to be helped to appreciate that the children too will have stories to tell. Showing the children memorabilia, as in the previous example of the playgroup children, can be very helpful and also any photographs of themselves as children at various ages, as these can provide an intriguing starting point for conversations.

Relationships take time to develop, so a number of contacts are usually more productive than a single visit. Children as well as elders need help in preparing the topics or themes to be covered during a visit or preferably a series of visits. Early productive topics in addition to schooldays could include childhood games, holidays and outings, favourite toys and technology. Early involvement in an activity that involves pairs or small groups working together, as in unpacking a memory box, viewing a short film and spontaneously continuing the story, dramatising the stories, drawing, or shared craft work, builds trust and mutual confidence.

Projects often begin with very modest objectives but, as people begin to enjoy their involvement, ideas develop and valued relationships, new knowledge, interesting activities and tangible and intangible benefits emerge. Plays, musicals, exhibitions, events, outings, visits, entertainments, published stories, books and poems as well as conventional and email correspondence, friendships, increased understanding and shared respect have all developed out of intergenerational work.

The children will need to plan and prepare for receiving their guests. They will need to courteously welcome their visitors, provide refreshments if possible, show the older people around the classroom and ensure they have somewhere comfortable to sit. The children too will need to practise asking questions beforehand, by interviewing each other and by learning to use open-ended questions instead of closed questions to explore agreed themes. Learning to listen carefully and remembering accurately is important. Children may also need to practise note taking and using a tape or digital recorder, camera or video camera. With very young children parents may be recruited as note takers. The classroom meeting then becomes a catalyst for further classroom activities of many different kinds. Follow-up visits to enable the children to display their work and convey their thanks are much appreciated.

Many schools and colleges are increasingly requiring senior students to engage in community service, either as part of the citizenship curriculum or as a requirement of educational qualifications such as the International Baccalaureate. The presence of older people in the classroom can permeate the whole curriculum. History, citizenship, language and literature, technology, geography, economics, nutrition, drama, art and music, social skills, religious education, values and morality are all areas of study that can benefit from intergenerational exchanges. Various interests, ambitions and aspirations can therefore be met by voluntary service to other people, including older people. Opportunities to undertake individual attachments focused on life story work, reminiscence or oral history are frequently sought and can prove mutually beneficial providing there is unambiguous agreement about the purpose, duration and content of what is intended and adequate preparation, training and oversight are in place.

Risk taking in intergenerational reminiscence projects

Embarking on intergenerational projects requires a careful assessment of risks and opportunities, as it is essential that neither older nor younger people be put at risk or hurt in any way in the process. Organisations intending to embark on intergenerational work must be sure to adhere to the relevant legal procedures concerned with safeguarding children and vulnerable adults and allow sufficient time for all relevant people, salaried staff and volunteers, to be vetted. Table 10.1 summarises the possible gains and losses that might be involved for participants of all ages.

Table 10.1: Opportunities and risks for participants in intergenerational reminiscence projects	
Opportunities	**Hazards and risks**
Relationship building through developing familiarity and trust – becoming friends	Increasing suspicion and distrust – alienation between older and younger people
Challenging age-related stereotypes	Confirming age-related stereotypes
Teaching the lessons of life-wisdom sharing	Rejecting the lessons of life
Transmitting cultural knowledge and history	Denying or rejecting cultural inheritance
Providing a role model	Rejecting of role model
Learning about contemporary life, interests, aspirations and experience	Lack of interest in learning about other's issues and concerns

If older people's recalled memories are not affirmed but instead are ignored or disregarded, denied or dismissed because they do not coincide with the dominant popularly accepted interpretation of history or are alien to the current concerns of society, this can be damaging and diminish well-being. This may happen, for example, if the prevailing collective view of wartime does not coincide with the personal experience of the individual. Thomson (2006), an oral historian, illustrates this important point when he describes the feelings of alienation of war veterans whose personal experience as combatants did not coincide with populist notions of glorious patriotic national achievements. Els van Dongen (2005, p.525), an anthropologist, writes about the predicament of older black disadvantaged South Africans who in the Apartheid era experienced violence, inequality and extreme poverty:

> Older people's memories of these experiences are not valued... memories, rather than bringing the generations together, have the opposite effect and widen the gap in understanding between the older and younger generations... the silencing of memories reflects the society's radical break with the past, which has made it difficult for younger people to mourn or sympathise with older people's losses.

This contrasts starkly with other South African oral history projects that are actively soliciting people's memories, sometimes as family projects, and preserving and archiving the stories in many different formats (Denis and Makiwane 2003). If problems associated with intergenerational sharing are encountered, whether in community-based groups, care facilities or families, alternative opportunities for elders to share their stories with fellow sufferers or with other receptive listeners must be generated.

It is equally important that the contributions of younger participants in intergenerational projects are also appreciated and that they too feel valued and respected. Although there are many potential hazards, many impressive gains have been reported in a growing literature concerned with intergenerational work which frequently includes a reminiscence dimension, although other objectives and outcomes may also be involved.

When recounting their own experience and values older people, although not infallible, need to be recognised as the 'experts'. This increases their self-esteem as they see themselves valued, respected and appreciated by the children. Each group learns from the other and, if working side by side over several weeks, older people develop greater awareness of modern educational methods, requirements, targets, testing, pressures and expectations which contemporary teachers and children face. This experience promotes their further recall and reconstruction of memories; it encourages the older informants to re-evaluate the past while at the same time their sympathies are enlarged towards modern children and young people. Frequently this results in a more balanced reappraisal of their past and present lives, few continuing to assert uncritically that 'it was better in my day'.

Underlying principles of intergenerational work in schools
Careful preparation of everyone involved has already been stressed. Separate preparation of both older and younger people is crucial to success. Only when each group has faced their apprehensions and shared their reservations will they be ready for meeting each other. Preliminary exercises that promote exploration of stereotypes usually assist with each group beginning to develop trust and willingness to move into joint meetings.

Locating interested older people requires time and effort in approaching local seniors' clubs, day centres, churches, temples and mosques, residential care facilities and sheltered housing. Build on existing relationships to open up possibilities for developing a collaborative project and in joint meetings identify the mutual objectives, anticipated gains and possible obstacles for older and younger groups.

Brief older participants on child protection issues and have an explicitly agreed protection policy in place which must be implemented meticulously. Listening carefully to a young person's opinions, concerns and feelings, without judging, can generate a lifeline to self-respect. It can provide much needed encouragement that the young person may otherwise lack.

Teaching skills for living through shared involvement

Older people's participation in classroom storytelling and writing projects encourages reflecting, sharing and writing by young children. According to Stelson and Dauk-Bleess (2003), elementary school teachers believe that 'shared projects can change the lives of children, deepen the community spirit of the classroom and expand empathy beyond the classroom walls' (p.40). They begin such writing projects by encouraging the children to brainstorm memories with an older partner and to jot down as many different memories as possible. The children then select three possibilities from their lists by asking themselves a series of reflective questions:

- Which experience can I see like a movie?
- Can I remember how I felt at the time?
- Am I willing to re-live the experience?
- Am I willing to make the memory public?
- Which memory says 'write about me'?

The children next try to recapture the intensity of the memories by briefly telling the three stories to their older partner who asks the child 'What is the hotspot of the story?' and 'Why is this experience important to you?' This process helps the child to choose the story he or she is willing to 're-live on paper' and the actual story writing begins. Through this staged process of recalling memories the children are helped to learn a structure and a method for future narrative writing and reflection. These children are beginning to learn in childhood how to recall, recapture and reappraise memories of their life experience rather than waiting until late life to begin to acquire these skills.

Minority ethnic community groups have much to contribute to school-based intergenerational work. Having older people from different cultural and religious traditions share their knowledge about their countries of origin, traditions, religion and culture, particularly if enriched by the display of memorabilia, artefacts, food and music, dramatically transforms lessons.

Many different intergenerational projects, whether in schools, youth groups, sports clubs or faith communities, can encourage and reinforce reminiscing and storytelling within families or compensate to some extent for its absence, thereby helping to develop children and young people's sense of identity and self-esteem – essential dimensions of successful life-long development.

Projects with older people located within health and social care facilities

These also have much to commend them but they 'feel' very different from school-based or youth club-based work. Here it is more difficult to develop true mutuality as the older people are likely to be physically or mentally frail, or both, much less independent and more likely to confirm younger people's stereotypical ideas of being old and outside the mainstream of life. The environment will suggest less mutuality and is likely to encourage any latent tendencies in the young people to bestow their beneficence rather than becoming mutual partners in a shared enjoyable enterprise. They may tend to see themselves as doing good, as entertainers rather than learners. Engagement in shared creative activities is the secret of successful work. With careful preparation and skilled implementation prior stereotypes held by both groups can be replaced by greater openness, mutual appreciation and genuinely shared pleasure (Gilfoy and Knocker 2008).

Grandparent involvement

Many schools run grandparent projects and where children do not have grandparents they are encouraged to involve other older relatives, neighbours or friends. Face to face contact is recommended but email and Internet usage now overcome some of the disadvantages associated with modern dispersed nuclear families. In these sorts of family projects children are usually set the task of interviewing the grandparents outside school hours. This approach is more akin to oral history projects in which semi-structured questions designed to gather information relating to particular topics or themes are used for a clearly defined purpose. They are more focused and more likely to elicit limited knowledge about lifetime experiences rather than prompt the child to appreciate the personal values of the older person. Such interviews, however, provide opportunities for children and their grandparents to develop greater trust and appreciation of each other with renewed, revitalised or enriched family contacts resulting. Teachers and parents need also to be sensitive to the risk that such projects may also pose for children who have fractured family relationships, or the absence or loss of older family members, which in small measure can be compensated for by using 'proxy' older people.

Visiting classrooms, watching short history films together and joining in the ensuing discussion is always productive. Audio and video recordings, photographs and published reminiscence accounts provide an excellent basis for creative writing, music and drama. Using one person's life story to develop awareness of social and economic changes over time provides a focused appreciation of personal experience located within a wider historical context. Unpacking memory boxes together and using local older people as guides for visits, excursions or trips to local historical sites and museums introduces varied personal points of view.

Having older people from ethnic minorities serve as culturally sensitive informants assists understanding of distant places as well as life in local ethnic communities. They can speak authentically about their different backgrounds and the experience of discrimination and cultural misunderstandings. Skills for life can be learned from authentic accounts of domestic life, work and working conditions, transport, medical services and many other topics. These can be explored productively in myriad ways when older and younger people of all ages share their ideas together (Strong 2010).

For children and grandchildren of immigrants, a sense of personal and community history is especially important in building self-esteem. 'Older people have a very positive role to play here, re-enforcing a cultural legacy, passing on personal stories and customs, and stimulating children in their communities to be interested in their own family histories' Schweitzer 2004, p.39).

'I was there when...' brings history alive. It transports us to another time and place. We hear a first-hand witness telling us how it was – and we are intrigued, fascinated, hooked and moved beyond our wildest imaginings. As past times come alive, either by first-hand accounts or by personal associations, we are informed and excited, sometimes with unexpected consequences as a community librarian co-facilitating an intergenerational group explains:

> Another member shared a letter he had found belonging to his grandmother. It was about how Queen Elizabeth II had distributed fruit baskets after her wedding so as not to waste all the fruit she had been given. This was a very welcome gesture in times of rationing. The letter which went with the basket caused a great stir in our group. It said 'Many kind friends overseas sent gifts of food at the time of my wedding. I want to distribute it as best I can, and to share my good fortune with others. I therefore ask you to accept this parcel with my very best wishes. Elizabeth.' The story however didn't end there. This gentleman sent a copy of the letter to Buckingham Palace and received a request asking if they could borrow it, as they didn't have an original copy in their archives. They wanted to display it at the summer opening of an exhibition in the State Rooms in Buckingham Palace, called A Royal Wedding. He agreed to the letter being retained in the Royal Archive and was delighted when he received a copy of *Five Gold Rings: A Wedding Souvenir Album from Queen Victoria to Queen Elizabeth II* and an invitation to attend the Palace to view the exhibition. On his visit, he was thrilled to see his grandmother's letter in pride of place displayed beside Queen Elizabeth's wedding dress and Prince Philip's uniform. (Quinn 2010, p.22)

A different approach to intergenerational reminiscence is illustrated by the 'Young Da Project' in Londonderry where the staff, together with older volunteer men who act as mentors, use reminiscence and life review techniques to encourage individuals, pairs and small groups of young fathers aged 14–25 to relate and review their life stories. This re-evaluation is encouraged as one means of assisting the young men to develop effective ways of conducting their lives and relationships. The life review discussions introduced by using lifelines form part of a broader programme of remedial, vocational and DIY education, study trips and life-enhancing recreational and educational experiences which are designed to assist the young men to develop skills for living, parenting and improving their economic, social and family prospects. (See www.da-youngfathersproject.co.uk.)

The promotion of intergenerational work

In recent years intergenerational work has emerged as an area of public policy interest in many western countries. This has developed partly as a response to the ageing of populations worldwide, recognition of the increasing role of grandparents as either primary or secondary carers due to family breakdown, death or absence of natural parents, and increasing interest in mobilising volunteers and in promoting a society for all ages. In the UK the Centre for Intergenerational Practice 'aims to support the development and promotion of intergenerational practice as a catalyst for social change'. It works in collaboration with the National Youth Agency and can be accessed at www.centreforip.org.uk. It also supports the International Consortium of Intergenerational Practice which holds biennial conferences, provides advice, publishes information and produces a journal. Issues such as the nature and identity of intergenerational work, clarifying relevant knowledge and methodologies and assuring standards in training and practice are all ongoing concerns.

Conclusion

This chapter and the two previous ones are concerned with encouraging people of different ages, backgrounds and circumstances to use their memories of past times, places, people and events for crossing boundaries and lessening the distance between themselves and other people. Although differences can divide, we are united by our common humanity if only we are confident to embrace it. Such confidence does not deny or fear difference. On the contrary reminiscence and recall seek to celebrate difference but also to discover shared experience in order more confidently to foster mutual respect between the generations, community solidarity and social inclusion. The past then provides a bridge to the present and a means for creating opportunities for helping people of all ages and diverse backgrounds to live peaceably together.

Key points

- Intergenerational work takes place in many different formal and informal settings including schools, colleges, youth groups, community arts and older people's groups, faith communities and health and social care services and it can involve children, young people and older people of varied ages.
- It requires meticulous separate and joint preparation of everyone involved.
- It is best spread out over a number of sessions or meetings to enable relationships to grow and practical work of many different kinds to be developed, shared, enjoyed, displayed and celebrated.

Application exercises

1. Explore the possibility of initiating an intergenerational reminiscence project. Identify possible objectives, participants, partners, likely gains, risks and outcomes.

2. As part of an intergenerational project ask a small group of older people to reminisce about themselves when young. Invite them to identify and list their teenage hopes and fears and then to suggest what they think the hopes and fears of contemporary teenagers might be. In a separate group ask teenagers to identify their own hopes and fears. Then bring both groups together to compare and contrast the three lists.

3. List what would encourage or discourage you from embarking on an intergenerational project.

Further reading

Golden, S. and Perlstein, S. (2004) *Legacy Works: Transforming Memory into Visual Art.* New York: Elders Share the Arts.

Hatton-Yeo, A. (2009) *Intergenerational Programmes: An Introduction and Examples of Practice.* Stoke-on-Trent: Beth Johnson Foundation.

International Consortium (2006) *International Practice, Policy and Performance: A Framework for Local Authorities.* Stoke-on-Trent: Beth Johnson Foundation.

Langford, S. and Mayo, S. (2001) *A Handbook of Intergenerational Arts: Sharing the Experience.* London: Magic Me.

Perlstein, S. and Bliss, J. (2003) *Generating Community: Intergenerational Partnerships through the Expressive Arts.* New York: Elders Share the Arts.

Chapter 11

Reminiscence with People with Dementia and Their Carers

Learning outcomes

After studying this chapter you should be able to:

- understand about the complexity of dementing conditions
- realise how dementia impacts on the person with dementia, their family and paid carers
- improve communication and build relationships with people with dementia by adapting and using reminiscence skills
- appreciate the similarities and differences between reminiscence, reality orientation, cognitive exercise and validation therapy
- undertake dementia-specific reminiscence and life story work with individuals, families and small groups affected by dementia.

Understanding dementia

Family and professional carers, friends and neighbours all find that dementia stretches their understanding, patience, perseverance and love. Dementia challenges us to find ways or re-discover old ways of staying in touch, in relationship, of continuing to communicate, because the person who develops dementia still remains a person who requires love, concern and respect. Too often pessimism, stigma, fatigue and fear leave people with dementia and their family carers unsupported and increasingly isolated as deterioration inevitably increases and dependency grows.

'Dementia' is an umbrella term for a syndrome that refers to a collection of progressive organic diseases of the brain, not to a single disease, which, while usually sparing physical health, affects cognitive, emotional and social aspects of functioning (Milwain 2009, 2010a, b and c). In its later stages physical functions are also seriously compromised. The symptoms include progressive inability to undertake the ordinary affairs of daily life because of severe and progressive decline in memory, reasoning, comprehension, learning capacity, judgement and problem solving. Social behaviour, emotional control, language, orientation and vitality are usually affected and depression and anxiety are also common. Dementia is not an inevitable consequence of ageing and is different from age-related minor forgetfulness. Most, but not all, dementias overtake people in later life. A small number of people, however, develop dementia in mid-life, or even earlier. The chances of being affected increase considerably from approximately three in every hundred people over 65 years of age to between ten and fifteen in every hundred people over 80 (Burns, Dening and Lawlor 2002).

Definitions, diagnosis, assessment and treatment are not standardised although the National Dementia Strategy covering England and Wales (DoH 2009a) and subsequent implementation guidance (DoH 2009b) provide strategy guidance that is gradually achieving improved health and social care provision for people with dementia, although much remains to be done throughout all parts of the UK. There is no definitive diagnostic test (except at post-mortem) although imagining procedures and accurate history taking coupled with close observation are considerably improving diagnosis and assessment. It remains difficult to calculate accurately the number of people with dementia. At present some 35 million people worldwide are thought to have dementia with this number doubling every 20 years. In the UK it is estimated that some 750,000 people, of which 16,000 are under 65, have dementia and it is anticipated that this number is likely to increase to one million by 2025 (Alzheimer's Society 2010). The numbers are steadily growing because, as more people live longer, the risk of developing dementia increases. Dementia has now become one of the major public health issues of the twenty-first century which costs the UK alone some £20 billion each year (Alzheimer's Society 2010; Knapp and Prince 2007). Dementia occurs in all countries and affects people regardless of gender, social class, income and ethnic group although it has been suggested that a higher level of education and continuing physical, social stimulation and possibly cognitive exercise offer some protection.

Research into the causes of dementia continues. Although various factors are implicated in the neurological deterioration which occurs, how any one person is affected depends on a complicated mix of physical factors, life experience, psychological factors (including unresolved past trauma), social relationships, emotional security and present circumstances (Kitwood 1997). It is possible to have more than one type of dementia simultaneously and diagnostic distinctions between different types are not always clear cut. Drugs that improve some people's symptoms and well-being at least for a time are now available so that early diagnosis to gain access to these treatments and to other supportive services is vital.

Alzheimer's disease is the most common dementia and often people use this term loosely to refer to all dementias, no matter what their type or cause. Alzheimer's disease and Lewy bodies dementia have no known cure, the cause is uncertain, the progression variable. Alzheimer's is estimated as accounting for 62 per cent of cases, vascular dementia for 17 per cent while 10 per cent of people with dementia have mixed dementia, 4 per cent Lewy bodies and 2 per cent fronto-temporal dementia including Pick's disease (Alzheimer's Society 2010). Vascular dementia is caused by repeated small strokes or haemorrhages in the brain. Preventive health measures like good diet and exercise throughout life and treatment for high blood pressure may assist prevention in some people to some extent. Other dementias include, among others, Korsakoff's linked to chronic alcoholism, AIDS, CJD, Parkinson's disease and stroke.

Person-centred care and person-in-relationship-centred approaches emphasise the importance of understanding the multiple factors, genetic and acquired, past and present, which contribute to any individual's unique pathway through the experience of dementia. There are neurological, psychological and social aspects to dementia that help to account for how different people are affected. As a progressive chronic terminal condition, usually lasting for many years, dementia makes heavy demands on family carers who are most often elderly spouses. Family carers are entitled to an assessment of their own needs and they will usually require information, respite and various domiciliary and supportive services as the demands made upon them change and increase over time (Nolan *et al.* 2006).

It is important, but not always easy, to distinguish dementia and depression as many of the symptoms seem to be similar. Depression frequently goes undiagnosed and untreated in older people. Depression in earlier life appears to increase the likelihood of dementia in later life while, for many people who have dementia, depression and anxiety are normal responses to these abnormal conditions. The memory and learning problems associated with dementia often resemble depression. Low mood, apathy, withdrawal and poor self-care seen in depression are also common in dementia. The ways in which mental and physical health are affected in dementia together with accompanying behavioural, mood and memory changes, and the speed of deterioration, vary greatly from person to person.

The term 'confusion' is often used instead of 'dementia'. Confusion is a symptom, rather than a disease. Many people with a dementing illness are indeed 'confused' about themselves, other people, where they are, and even the time of day. Except in the very advanced stages, people with dementia are seldom totally confused. They may be clear about some things and very mixed up about others. Some die early, others live for many years. Some people's behaviour may be very difficult and demanding, beyond their control. Yet there are others who, if treated in ways that meet their individual needs for care, attachment, security, respect and freedom from stress, are able to function reasonably well long into their illness.

In the early stages of dementia, as people become increasingly aware of their failing memory, many feel anxious, agitated, restless and depressed. Other losses and life changes, especially losing a spouse or partner, or moving to an unfamiliar environment, will make their problems more visible and may also accelerate decline. As the disease develops, people find it hard, but not impossible, to learn new skills or information, to remember recent events or recall old information on demand, to hold a coherent conversation, and to manage personal and domestic affairs, including personal hygiene. They may be unaware of danger, get lost in familiar places or be unable to make decisions or to plan ahead. At times their behaviour can cause embarrassment and offence. As the disease progresses they are likely to grow more withdrawn and isolated, cut off from others, who may be slow to realise initially that something is seriously wrong.

Often relatives, friends and neighbours feel that the person who has early dementia is just being difficult. As deterioration continues, both professional and family carers need to find ways of dealing with their own anxiety – will I go the same way? It is crucial for family and professional carers to develop their abilities to continue to relate to the person with dementia as a real person, with real feelings, not just a dependent non-person needing only physical care. They must find ways of reinforcing the person's humanity, rather than undermine the already precarious sense of self. How others respond to those with dementia influences how the person sees him or herself which in turn influences behaviour, regardless of the underlying neurological damage.

Although sooner or later dementia affects all cognitive functions, it is short-term or working memory, often described as recent memory, that is first affected. Recall of more distant times, places and people, especially memories relating to significant personal life experience (episodic memory) and associated physical skills and actions (procedural memory), may remain relatively intact or partially intact far into the disease. Semantic memory refers to well-learned facts and acquired information and concepts which along with episodic memories related to specific places and situations will endure for a time but are eventually lost or evade recall. Autobiographical memories are long-term memories recalled by an individual. It is possible to assist people to key into early memories to some extent and use this recall to encourage conversation and stimulate individual and group activities and so preserve and enhance sociability. Multi-sensory triggers, prompts and sometimes personally significant surroundings can assist this process and thereby increase the well-being and care of people with mild, moderate and, to a limited extent, severe dementia (see also Chapters 5 and 6).

> ...for while my yesterdays
> Are strangely dim and shrouded in recall,
> The far back things are vivid to my gaze
> And joyous is my welcome to them all.

> (W.F. Marshall 1983, p.126)

The importance of having clear objectives

In planning reminiscence work with people with dementia and their carers, realistic goals that take account of the worker's own level of expertise, confidence, available assistance, access to supervision and the context in which the work is undertaken require careful consideration. Considerable sensitivity, empathy, patience and skill are necessary. The essential key is to be positive, to emphasise what the person with dementia can still do, and not what is now difficult or impossible. The guidance given in earlier chapters is also relevant but needs to be substantially modified when identifying and responding to the needs and interests of people with dementia and their carers. Objectives usually emphasise:

- increasing sociability and lessening isolation by preserving and developing personal relationships
- having fun and encouraging communication
- providing social and intellectual stimulation by exercising retained abilities
- decreasing boredom by involvement in creative reminiscence-related activities
- preserving a sense of identity and self-esteem
- reducing anxiety and contributing to well-being
- sustaining family and paid carers, and developing their understanding and skills
- informing assessments and care plans.

Reminiscence workers with professional training are also using reminiscence in systematic structured life reviews, counselling and psychotherapy with people who have dementia whose behaviour is troubled and troubling or who have low mood, depression or problematic or intrusive memories.

Supporting carers

Many family and paid carers find dementia care exceedingly stressful, even if rewarding in some ways. Without adequate support systems, it may become overwhelming. Mutual involvement in reminiscence makes it easier to concentrate effort on what people can still do, rather than being overwhelmed by what they can no longer do. Reminiscence is a relatively low risk, easily managed, cheap, enjoyable, effective psycho-social intervention which also gives carers pleasure and satisfaction. It helps prevent setting the person with dementia up for failure by making unrealistic, stressful demands on their failing short-term memory and other compromised abilities because it principally relies on long-term memory.

Family carers, professional carers and reminiscence workers are often surprised at how well people with mild to moderate dementia can reminisce. Even in later stages when the response seems small and transitory judged by 'ordinary' standards, it can still give great mutual pleasure to the person and the carer by helping to hold both in warm, loving relationships (Schweitzer and Bruce 2008).

Communicating with people with dementia

> What have I got to tell them? Stories!
>
> And nobody asks, so I don't bother telling them.
>
> (Killick' 2005)

The failure too often rests with the carer who grows weary of making the effort to communicate. Professional and family carers need to develop ways of communicating that respect the person and reach beyond ordinary speech. This is not always easy to do but Goldsmith (1996) argues that it is possible to learn to communicate with people with dementia. It requires great patience, time and empathy – a willingness to try to see the world through their eyes, rather than through our own, to walk in their shoes or sit in their chair (Kitwood 1997). By careful listening to conversation about the past the person can be appreciated, as he or she used to be and now is. Positive attitudes and willingness to try to talk and to listen are far more important than a list of techniques. Abandon expectations that people with dementia should be able to converse as they used to if only they would try harder; they have changed and so must carers – the 'well' person must take responsibility for initiating and persevering in encouraging communication by every possible means (Killick and Allan 2001).

Non-verbal communication – reading and responding to body language

Everyone, with or without dementia, uses both words and body language to communicate. When brain damage, regardless of its cause, disrupts verbal language, skill in reading non-verbal body language becomes crucial. Body language refers to body movements, big or small, facial expression, eye movements, touch, physical appearance, posture, gesture, demeanour, and use of personal space or positioning. Verbal communication refers to pitch, intonation and rate of speaking as well as to content of speech. In dementia there may be vague and inaccurate or jumbled speech, diminished or impoverished vocabulary, changes in word association patterns, difficulty in finding words, repetition, slowness of response and disordered or disjointed conversation. While it is crucial to listen carefully and try to unravel or decode the meanings of words and associated emotions, it is just as important to encourage non-verbal expression through gestures, mime, actions or demonstrations, and to become skilled in 'reading' this form of communication. Here are some simple tips, that may also be relevant to communication with people who have other types of learning, visual, hearing or speech difficulties. Techniques like these can help but only if there is genuine regard and respect for the person with dementia who will usually be very perceptive about how others feel towards them. Accurate observation, patience, slowed pace and empathy are the keys to good communication. 'Good care is slow care' sums up this advice.

Setting the scene

- Check the basics. Spectacles need to be clean and of the right prescription, hearing aids properly fitted and functioning with live batteries, and dentures in place.
- Do not compete with other distractions, especially radio, television or others' competing conversations. If necessary move to another quiet room. Many older people find it very difficult and often extremely uncomfortable to cope with competing sources of sound.

- Meet in a well-lit room with the light coming from behind and do not cover your mouth. Older people require greater light illumination than younger people.
- Eye contact is always important when either speaking or listening (providing this is not impolite in the person's original culture).
- Sit at the same level as the other person.
- Attract the person's attention before speaking, make eye contact, smile and nod encouragement.
- Relax and concentrate, focusing attention on the other person, and listen attentively in a calm and unhurried way.

Interactions

- Take the initiative in beginning a conversation. People with dementia find it hard to get started and usually take time to 'warm up'.
- Remain still. Moving around or changing places can be a distraction.
- If a person is restless, possibly link arms and walk together, but talking while walking may not be easy.
- Speak slowly and clearly but never in a childish way. Do not talk down to people and never talk over their heads to someone else.
- Do not try to correct the person. Do not argue. Accept what is said.
- Slow down, take your time and give the person time to gather their thoughts together and time to respond.
- If workers are hurried and tense, there is every possibility that the person with dementia will sense this.
- Appear relaxed – adopting a relaxed posture helps the body to relax.
- Use short sentences. If asking questions, these should be simple and direct. Ask only one question at a time. Open-ended questions are usually more productive.
- Try rephrasing if not at first understood, always using low and not high-pitched tones. Encourage actions, mime and demonstration. Take care to check whether the person may also have a hearing impairment so appropriate assistance is received. (See also Chapter 13.)

- Respond to the person's underlying emotions and intended communication, as best understood, rather than being preoccupied with factual accuracy.
- Finding the correct word may be difficult – a person might use one word when another is meant, so be open to various interpretations.
- Use encouraging smiles and nods.
- At times it may be helpful to use touch if this seems acceptable.
- Laughter binds people together. Humour endures despite dementia. Shared pleasure (and tears), even without words, bring people closer.

(Harris 2006, p.125) quotes Brooker, a psychologist, who described communication with people with dementia as 'like a game of tennis, with a message rather than a ball being batted backwards and forwards'. The carer's task is to coach, not to win. Preparation is essential so the worker can create the best conditions to capture the person's attention as well as lobbing the ball with the best chance of a successful return so that both enjoy the conversation.

If a person with dementia is to undertake a task, it helps to analyse it so it can be broken down into separate small steps which can then be presented one at a time in the correct sequence. This way there is a better chance of the person being able to perform the task. Give warm praise and encouragement. Never use negative examples or critical responses to reinforce a point and concentrate on what a person can still do rather than on what they can no longer do.

As dementia progresses a person is liable eventually to reach the point where he or she can no longer remember the detail of their own story. They then need someone else to hold the story for them or, put another way, to become the custodian of the story. The Beirut hostage Brian Keenan (2009, p.233) recalls how his mother's memories became so disjointed as she journeyed further and further into Alzheimer's and how urgent it became for him to recover and store the fragments:

> Sometimes she pretended to remember, to avoid the struggle. What remained were like fragments of an old faded cine film. Lots of times the reel of memory came to a flickering stop, only to restart again several years later.

Reminiscence is one imaginative means that can be used to lay down a story store which can then be used to prompt the owner in ways which help stave off social isolation, lowered self-esteem and threatened identity.

Loss of memory does not automatically mean loss of creativity or capacity to feel and to express empathy. Music, movement, mime, touch, dance, drama and art can all be used, or used in conjunction with reminiscence. Indeed it is essential that people with dementia continue to have opportunities to express their creativity, for as Cohen (2004) argues persuasively creativity, for everyone as they age strengthens their morale, contributes to physical health, enriches relationships and serves to provide a legacy.

Rather than thinking the seemingly garbled, often repetitive talk of people with dementia is meaningless, some professional and family carers are learning to 'read', unravel and respond to the symbolism, metaphor and emotional content of the words used. Killick (1994, p.16), a poet, listens very attentively to people with dementia, recording their conversations which he crafts into poetry to give back to the person. He explains it in this way:

> It seems to me that language used by people with dementia is a metaphorical one – where what they say often does not make sense in the usual literal way but has a poetic or symbolic meaning. People express themselves in language nearer to poetry than they used before. For example, one lady talked about her experience as a monkey puzzle, and another expressed a yearning for freedom as riding on a swing.

Sometimes the conversation refers to the past; sometimes to poignant, insightful comment on the present. Here are two poems from Killick's book *You Are Words: Dementia Poems* (1997, p.10 and p.39) which illustrate these points.

> *You Are Words*
> Life is a bit of a strain,
> in view of what is to come.
> Sometimes I feel embarrassed
> talking to anybody, even you.
> You don't really like to burden
> other people with your problems.
> I have been a strict person.

What people and children do now
is completely different. Any beauty
or grace has been desecrated.
The circle of life is shot away.
I want to thank you for listening.
You see, you are words.
Words can make or break you.
Sometimes people don't listen,
they give you words back,
and they're all broken, patched up.
But will you permit me to say
that you have the stillness of silence,
that listens and lasts.

Grass
A young fella carried me
in here; it were a long way
and a long time ago.
I were lying on grass...
I don't want to stay, no
there's nothing for me
they're all very kind
but I don't want to be
inside anywhere at all
it's much too hot and bright
it just don't feel right
I've not been used
I need the fresh air
I keep calling out;
Nurse, Nurse, carry me
outside to where
I were lying on grass.

Special places and spaces which encourage reminiscence

In addition to these creative ways of reaching out to people with dementia, the physical design of care facilities can assist or detract from effective dementia care. Marshall (1998) describes internationally accepted principles of design for dementia. A building needs to have its own integrity so that its parts promote easy recognition of the diverse functions performed in various spaces. Décor and furnishings of some parts of a building and its surroundings are sometimes deliberately designed, however, to resemble times past and thus promote opportunities for enjoyable recall. Outdoor spaces and gardens, for example, which utilise old-fashioned familiar perfumed plants, shrubs, trees and vegetables, together with artefacts and sociable sitting and activity areas with safe wandering paths, are increasingly used. Dedicated rooms furnished according to the times when present residents were teenagers and young to middle-aged adults are becoming popular. One residential care worker said:

> I furnished a room in our home as a kitchen-house. Walking into it with a resident is like walking into their past. We have another room furnished as a pub with old-fashioned beer mats, bottles, photos and furniture. In here the men tell many a yarn over a pint of Guinness.

Develop the habit of thinking systematically about making use of the natural and designed environment to mark different stages of people's life journeys and the places and people that were and possibly still may be important to them. In ever widening circles beginning with a person's bedroom, then moving outwards to their current care home, neighbourhood and community, identify cherished possessions, significant landmarks and sacred places which can be used as way markers, signposts and hooks on which to hang present conversations. Trips or pilgrimages to once significant familiar places can be richly rewarding for older people with dementia as well as their family and professional carers.

Guidance for planning dementia-specific reminiscence groups

Deciding whether to do individual work or group work will depend upon the persons involved, the context in which you are working and the objectives you wish to achieve. Group work with people with dementia is not only possible but is very rewarding, providing groups are small – probably with no more than two to four members, who must be selected with great care. Such small groups enable each member actively to participate and to feel that they and their contributions are valued. Remember that many older people with dementia are also likely to have sensory impairments that may hinder participation in a group. Some people will prefer the personal, undivided attention that individual work provides.

Many, however, enjoy the sociability of a small group that can counteract the encroaching isolation caused by memory loss and associated language difficulties. In a small intimate group where people feel relaxed and appreciated, they often rediscover the rules of conversation such as turn taking, listening to others and responding warmly to other people's contributions. The gains from mixing in a small group must be balanced with the problem many people with Alzheimer's have of keeping track of who said what in a group conversation so that special care is required when selecting potential participants.

In small numbers people with dementia can also participate successfully in groups where the majority of members do not have obvious memory difficulties. Depending on individual circumstances segregation in dementia-specific groups is not always necessary. Successful membership of a heterogeneous group can be stimulating and rewarding providing the other members are encouraging and tolerant.

The general advice already given about excluding people with particular kinds of problems from groups also applies to those who have dementia (see Chapter 5). Do not include anyone in a group who is likely to harm another member or make it difficult for others to participate comfortably.

Even in a very small group it is helpful to have two facilitators in order to give personal attention, to share tasks and to cope if anyone becomes upset or wishes to leave the group. With more helpers, groups can be enlarged and effectively use a mixture of paired, small group and whole group activities.

Remembering Yesterday, Caring Today (RYCT) projects

Larger groups with up to 20 people have been used very successfully in Remembering Yesterday, Caring Today (RYCT) projects pioneered by the European Reminiscence Network. These time-limited groups consist of people with dementia, their family carers, volunteers and leaders drawn from various health, social care and artistic backgrounds. RYCT groups combine richly varied shared reminiscence activities which emphasise the creative arts. The groups provide opportunities for having fun together, breaking down barriers, learning and re-learning to communicate, enhancing relationships and encouraging sociability. Bruce, Hodgson and Schweitzer's (1999) RYCT handbook available in a number of European languages together with Schweitzer and Bruce's (2008) *Remembering Yesterday, Caring Today* give detailed guidance about how to run RYCT groups and particularly how to manage paired, small group and whole group activities within sessions. A large UK multi-centre randomised controlled trial of the effectiveness of the RYCT approach for people with dementia and their carers is currently being undertaken; its analysis of outcomes is awaited with considerable interest.

Obtaining consent

Obtaining consent is important, but not always easy to achieve. Always extend a brief, honest invitation, supplemented by a simple written explanation. Encourage people to attend, remind them on the day and be finely tuned to non-verbal signs of pleasure or distress. Let them try it out to see if they like it as it may be difficult for them to understand what is meant by reminiscence. Make it possible for people to indicate in whatever way they are able if they do not wish to participate. It is best to leave the door of the meeting room ajar; do not prevent anyone leaving if they so wish but make sure they are accompanied if there is likely to be any risk involved.

If a person comes, remains and appears to enjoy the experience, their assent may be taken as consent. It is advisable, although not strictly necessary, to secure the consent of principal relatives and to secure their cooperation whenever possible. Although most welcome the opportunity for involvement there may be someone who does not wish their family member to be involved in reminiscence (Hughes and Baldwin 2006).

Adapting style, pace and programme

Small formed groups that meet regularly for up to 20 sessions are more effective than groups which have fewer sessions or a shifting membership. If possible consider holding sessions more frequently than once a week. They should always be held in the same place, at the same time of day, and follow the same general pattern. Some workers like to provide familiarity and a sense of continuity by wearing the same clothes, perfume or after shave at each session. A regular structure or pattern to the group meeting is desirable. Identical opening and ending rituals, songs, greetings and goodbyes, using mascots, symbols and candles or simple actions such as joining hands can provide continuity, reminders and a sense of security, inclusion and familiarity.

Try to hold the group at the time of day when the members are more lucid. Careful observation will reveal what is their best time. As a rough general guide, many people with dementia seem to be more restless and disorientated in the late afternoon or twilight, perhaps because of altered visual cues caused by changing light and deepening shadows. Well-planned reminiscence held at this time of day can constructively occupy 'sundowners' and effectively counteract their anxious preoccupations over lost attachment figures by giving them undivided attention, distraction and reassurance.

A person with dementia cannot be expected to call up specific memories on demand. The worker has to set the scene and provide the relevant and appropriate stimuli. Sessions may need to be shorter than an hour but many people with mild to moderate dementia can retain interest far longer than is usually expected, provided the triggers and topics are relevant and the general ambience is congenial. If people get restless, adjust the programme. Switch to triggers that stimulate other senses or introduce another activity to match the mood of the members that will probably vary anyway within meetings and from meeting to meeting. Allow time for unhurried refreshments and a physical activity that translates recalled memories into physical, artistic or other creative formats by using simple drama, mime, singing, dance or art.

Multi-sensory triggers are especially important and they should closely relate to people's known background, previous interests and preferred sensory pathways. Do not overwhelm or overload people. Use triggers sparingly and selectively, usually one at a time and in sequence, so that all senses can be used as pathways to cognitive, emotional, physical and social stimulation.

It is very natural to combine reminiscing with other activities that depend on procedural long-term memory – memories of embodied actions because 'we remember through our bodies as much as through our nervous system and brain' and 'perception, memory and imagination are in constant interaction' (Pallasmaa 2005, p.50 and p.67). Make full use of humour and create opportunities for everyone to enjoy themselves, to be friends and to have a good time together (Heathcote 2007; Schweitzer 1998b).

Montessori methods in dementia care

Interesting parallels have been made between the Montessori approach to educating very young children and rehabilitating people with dementia by means of companionable engagement in long practised tasks that are recovered and reconstructed through reminiscence and recall as Brenner and Brenner (2004, p.25) suggest:

> If the Montessori activity is polishing silverware, a daughter might reminisce with her mother about dinners she served or parties they attended together. Working together on a meaningful project can give joy in the moment, and perhaps bring back shared joy from long ago.

These authors suggest that the Montessori principles on which this approach is based include:

- use of real life materials that are aesthetically pleasing
- progression from simple to complex, concrete to abstract
- materials and procedures structured so that participants can work from left to right, and from top to bottom
- materials arranged in order from largest to smallest, and from most to least
- learning progresses in an orderly sequence: participant watches presentation, tries replicating it and talks about the activity
- activities are broken into component parts, and one component is practised at a time
- the risk of failure is minimised, and chances of success are maximised
- as little vocalisation as possible is used when demonstrating activities
- participation is always invited and never enforced
- when presenting activities the speed of movement is slowed to match the speed of the participants
- wherever possible the materials and activity is made self-correcting

- whenever possible the participants are encouraged to create something that can be used by the larger community
- the environment is adapted to the needs of the participants
- whenever possible the participants select the activities.

With detailed knowledge of a person's background it is easy to see how these principles can incorporate a reminiscence dimension that is well matched to earlier life experience. In this way the Montessori goal of assisting people to become as independent as possible is encouraged.

Locating and using relevant triggers

Speak with older friends, relatives and others with local knowledge to discover what triggers relate to the past lives of the people who are to be involved in reminiscence. It is helpful if people's own personal possessions are available. It may be possible to borrow artefacts from places where people once worked or to find volunteers with similar work backgrounds who might join a group. It is an added bonus if the reminiscence workers and volunteers share the same background as members and speak in a familiar accent or idiom. As one day centre worker said:

> People with dementia come to our day centre for two days a week. It's in an area of the town where a lot of people live who once worked in the local mill so we have gathered up a lot of old bobbins, spools, wool and different types of cloth. We also have old newspapers with pictures of mills and mill workers, and our local museum gave us a recording of a mill hooter, a sort of siren that was blown at the start and end of the shift. We use all these things with two or three women together, or sometimes just with one person to get them talking.

Communicating through music

Music is especially effective for reaching people with dementia, but like all other interventions it must be used in a person-centred way. Aldridge (2000), a university teacher and researcher, suggests music serves many functions, including calming and comforting people who are agitated; reducing wandering; improving self-esteem; stimulating memories and emotions; connecting people; and lifting the spirit. Musical ability and musical appreciation appear to be retained long after other abilities have deteriorated. Some people with no evidence of prior musical ability or earlier musical training, given non-threatening opportunities to participate in music making and listening to music, do so with obvious pleasure.

Encourage people to play percussion instruments, sing along, tap their feet, sway, wave scarves, clap or dance. Words or fragments of once-loved songs and hymns may be sung, sometimes spontaneously, sometimes with prompting, even when ordinary speech has deteriorated. Live music evokes rich response and gives great pleasure. It may also trigger sad recollections. Take the trouble to discover what kind of music each person may have enjoyed and now prefers. Do not expect everyone to share the same tastes and ask relatives if they can provide previously loved tapes or CDs. Music combined with physical movement such as dance or used together with other methods of sensory stimulation has proved effective. Simpler, slower and clearer melodies may come to be appreciated as much as old favourites (Clair 1996). (See also Chapter 6.)

A nurse describes how:

> It was as a student nurse on my first ward that I first looked after an Alzheimer's patient. Mrs Smith was loud and it was impossible to have a conversation with her. She had a tendency to be violent, was agitated and she would not eat or drink. I started singing to her. At first she did not respond at all, but after a short time she began to join in. Not only did she know the words of all the songs but she had a wonderful singing voice. This woman who could not speak a coherent sentence could sing perfectly.

Reminiscing with troubled individuals

In caring for particularly troubled and troubling individuals whose behaviour challenges others, specific reminiscence is well worth trying. Neurological deterioration, life experience, personality and present circumstances will all be implicated in contributing to disruptive behaviour. Because these troubled people create so many difficulties for everyone around – including other older people, family carers and paid carers as well as themselves – if life can be made better for them, it will also be better for everyone else. Unravelling the life story of troubled people enlarges the carer's understanding; such knowledge suggests possible explanations and points to possible constructive ways of responding. (See also Chapter 7.)

The importance of senior staff support

Too many group living facilities and day centres do not customarily provide opportunities for intensive attention to individuals although an activity programme based on group work may be in place. If specific reminiscence work is to be undertaken which involves giving more time and attention than is customary to a particular person, it is important for this to be noted in the care plan and fully explained to all staff, including administrative, care and domestic staff. Without such formal backing from managers, any worker asked to undertake specific reminiscence work with an individual risks being isolated, unsupported and even sabotaged. (Chapter 5 discusses the responsibilities of senior managers in providing vital support.)

If this support is not provided, other staff will criticise their colleague for neglecting ordinary duties and for paying too much attention to one person. The work attempted will be undermined if all staff members have not been persuaded that it is right to single out an individual for concentrated special attention. Work can be sabotaged in many different ways unless all staff members believe reminiscence and life story work are 'real work', as the following example from a research worker shows:

> Mary, a widow living in a care home, was selected for 'specific' reminiscence work. She was a most unhappy, isolated, aggressive, anorexic widowed woman who pushed, hit, spat and shouted at anyone who came near. The key worker collected a detailed life history from Mary's niece and discovered that, when younger, Mary had always liked nice things such as fine china, good linen and small delicate flowers.
>
> So the key worker decided to try to tempt her to eat by setting a breakfast tray with a linen tray cloth, special china and a posy of flowers. Mary started to eat better and some days she asked for a second piece of toast. Her aggression decreased and her isolation lessened. On the days when the key worker was off duty, the special arrangements were ignored because the cook refused to set the tray, so opposed was she to the idea of one resident being singled out for special attention. Several weeks passed before the officer in charge confronted the cook and instructed her not to undermine the care plan and to set the tray.

Observation

Specific work in a group care setting must begin with careful observation extending over several days. If the person with dementia resides at home the following advice will need to be adjusted somewhat. Managers must make it possible for the selected staff member to have time to carry out observations and to write a detailed care plan, which will need to be reviewed from time to time. This may mean allocating more staff time. But more often it means staff using time differently.

Such work is based on careful, precise observation of present behaviour and detailed life history information gathered from all available sources. This information is used to shed light on present behaviour. Observations should cover the daily pattern of life so as to identify any recurring positive or negative aspects and to detect any related events, circumstances and timings. Close detailed observation draws a picture of the person's present lifestyle. It is advisable to observe:

- times of the day or night when the person may be especially happy or unhappy, disturbed, troubled, restless or agitated
- time spent alone
- interactions with other residents or staff
- preferences for how and where the day is spent
- the relevance, responsiveness, appropriateness and content of speech and behaviour
- variations in mood, lucidity, activity and interests
- behaviour around major routines of the day such as getting up, bedtime, bathing, toileting and meal-time behaviour
- ability to manage self-care and other activities of daily living
- personal preferences for food, clothes, company and activities
- number of and reactions to visits by friends, family or volunteers.

Gathering life history details

Information about life history draws a picture of the person's past lifestyle that can then be used to help 'decode' the outcomes identified from observation of present behaviour. The life history connects people to the present. So many older people with dementia who live in care facilities resemble refugees. They are strangers in strange places, cut off from their past and alienated from the present. Life history, skilfully used, can link a distant past with a problematic present. It also enables carers to understand what may be troubling or unsettling a person in the present.

If the history depends only on what the person can tell about themselves, the past often remains shadowy, fragmented with just fleeting glimpses. Life story work, or structured life review, however, as described in Chapter 7, may be fruitful ways of gaining information which can then be added to by consulting relatives, contemporaries and agency records.

Too frequently these records give only negative accounts of recent or present functioning. They tend to be problem focused and emphasise physical symptoms. They stress what people can no longer do and say little about what capacities remain and what lifetime interests might be preserved or revived. Reminiscence workers and professional carers should try to imagine their own lives to date summarised in just a few lines on an assessment form supplemented by a plethora of tick boxes. This would not do justice to them at a much younger age. Yet this is often all that is known about the long lives of so many older people in hospitals, care homes or day centres (Bell and Troxel 1997, 2001).

Be sensitive but persistent in researching the life history. Search for clues about significant past events, people and places and possible present resource people. Be alert to the possibility that the origins of present behaviour may lie in unresolved past trauma, pain and loss which under the influence of dementia is leaking into the present. Never, however, dismiss the possibility that it could be aspects of the present care environment which are causing or aggravating the difficulties. Keep careful records of what information is gathered.

Useful information includes the following:

- important chronological events such as births, deaths and marriages
- information about parents
- childhood, school and student days
- spouses, partners, children and grandchildren
- family life and work
- significant friends and relationships
- significant pets and possessions

- major life crises or trauma, landmarks, changes or branching points and transitions
- where WWII was spent and how it was experienced
- places lived in or visited
- hobbies, interests, trips and preferred music and recreation.

Start reminiscing with the person. Learn to listen very attentively and respond to the expressed emotions while also picking up information. Some conversation may need to be decoded or translated. Listen for recurring themes or repeated words. Do not be preoccupied with establishing factual accuracy. Try to decipher the symbolic meanings and unravel allusions and metaphors. Begin by assuming truth rather than falsity, belief rather than disbelief, genuineness not confabulation.

Stop labelling people as 'confused' and dismissing muddled conversation as irrelevant, especially if a person is obviously upset, perhaps struggling to tell you about something that has caused them hurt in either the distant or recent past. Try to get sufficient clues to check the story out with someone who may remember something from the past that has now 'leaked' into the present.

All too often when a person with dementia is upset, tearful or distressed about a past memory which has intruded into the present, workers hastily change the conversation and attempt distraction or denial. Some may even physically or emotionally remove themselves from the conversation. Gradually reminiscence workers will find with practice that they are able to extend their ability to feel their way into the world of the other person with increasing willingness to explore past pain and share past sadness. As confidence grows they may be able to piece together the fragments of the story (possibly assisted by the life history details gathered from other sources) which is causing distress at the present time. The following example of Andy and Anna illustrates the need for this kind of detective work.

Social worker Andy, who used to be a sociable friendly man, had early-onset dementia. He had withdrawn into a world of silence, no longer even talking to his devoted wife who was determined to care for him at home. During a planned reminiscence session with him at a day centre when a collection of family photographs was being used to try to stimulate conversation, he was shown a picture of Niagara Falls. He launched at once into a long, apparently garbled tale about a woman who had thrown her baby over the Falls. The worker, thinking this was a bizarre fantasy, hastily changed the conversation. Later, when checking back with his wife, every detail as told by Andy was found to be correct.

Involving partners in reminiscence work

Older relatives, especially spouses and partners, are often delighted to be asked for information. They feel they are contributing to the care of their person who as the dementia progresses will inevitably change. Positive benefits for the partner from either parallel or joint reminiscence can also occur.

Yukiko Kurokawa (1998), a Japanese psychologist, describes ways of undertaking shared reminiscence work with couples when one has dementia. Unlike Barbara Haight's structured life review work described in Chapter 7 which is done strictly with the individual person, she facilitates a simultaneous joint life review, in which couples are helped to recall, share, review and integrate memories of shared life experience. She suggests that by this process the well spouse is better able to cope with the partner's deterioration and both partners enjoy re-living and integrating satisfying aspects of their past lives. This mutual journey is often given tangible form by creating a collage from personal photographs or, if these are unavailable, pictures from magazines chosen by the participants to capture mood as well as memories are used.

Making a plan

When the detailed life history has been gathered, make a written plan of how the information is to be used. The plan is only a guide to a possible journey the reminiscence worker and the person with dementia will take together. There will be unexpected detours, surprises, excitement, shared pleasure and, no doubt, some disappointments and possibly some shared tears as well. This is the beginning of a demanding journey because the worker has to be finely tuned to the present as well as to past history. It is essential not to lose sight of physical and emotional care needs related to the person's present care and well-being while becoming so absorbed in gathering the life story and the life history details.

Implementing the plan

Use the information to introduce focused conversation. Discuss cherished memorabilia, perhaps work on a life story book, go on trips, outings or visits to once-significant places, re-introduce old hobbies or follow up old interests, to rekindle further recall. The information collected will give clues to possible fruitful topics of conversation and enjoyable activities. Become an active proxy memory bank, holding the deposits on behalf of the person with dementia, drawing on the riches to benefit the owner who requires assistance to access them in the present.

When the conversation is set in safe territory, people may be sufficiently secure to risk responding. Ease them gently into situations and to conversations and activities that emphasise what they can still do. They may be well aware of their deficiencies and need warm, loving encouragement, time and patience to risk responding. Use life history to select triggers and arrange situations that resemble past experience. Helping with simple cooking, cleaning or laundry, trips to the seaside or parks and garden centres, a night at the greyhounds, a soccer match or an evening in the local pub can give immense pleasure to people with dementia. They can often 'pass' themselves in such situations without their dementia becoming apparent or socially inhibiting. Circumstances and surroundings, if sufficiently familiar, can stir long-dormant memories and well-learned behaviour. The experience is enjoyed at the time, but it also provides a focus for future recall, further conversation and recurring pleasure.

Reviewing the work undertaken
Always take stock of what work has been attempted. Workers should credit themselves for success and face up to failures. Such intensive work with individuals contributes to personal and professional development. It helps workers to grasp the uniqueness of each person and to understand how the past influences the present. It brings great mutual pleasure and increased job satisfaction when staff see evidence of their developing skills and deeper understanding which has contributed to improved well-being for individuals and for others around them.

Staff find they can cope better with troubled and troubling people by decreasing their isolation and lessening their unhappiness. Because this kind of individual work changes relationships and lessens the distance between staff and older people and their families, attitudes change, tolerance grows and sympathies are enlarged in ways which reduce the awfulness of dementia for all involved. (See Chapter 16 on staff development.) An officer in charge of a dementia- specific home described how:

> Elizabeth always disrupted meal times by shouting and messing with her food. Her detailed life history showed she had always preferred to lie in and rise late. Instead, our staff members were getting her up early, hurrying her to get dressed and to come downstairs for breakfast.
>
> We decided to be more relaxed. She was left to sleep until she woke. Her key worker then helped her dress at her own pace. By the time she came downstairs, most people had finished breakfast and Elizabeth could eat in solitude which seemed to suit her much better. Her shouting disappeared, she complained less about a sore back and she ceased to be a trouble to everyone else.

Disturbed reactions

Very occasionally, someone may have an over-reaction that is inappropriate to his or her present circumstances. This 'catastrophic reaction', a term now less used, is like an electric circuit becoming overloaded and an appliance blowing a fuse to avoid further damage. If this happens, try to stay calm; do not waste energy on trying to reason with the distressed person or talk them out of their exaggerated response. Gentle distraction and patience are more likely to be effective. A cup of tea together is an easy way of providing comforting reassurance. Try to keep life simple with gentle routines that provide order without rigidity; familiarity without monotony; occupation without pressure; and peacefulness without clamour. Do not take the upset personally but think about whether something done which in future could be avoided or current circumstances might have innocently provoked the unforeseen exaggerated outburst.

If something in a reminiscence session appears to trigger an eruption, avoid those particular triggers, topics or associations with the person in the future. The behaviour may be totally unrelated to the reminiscence work, so do not hastily conclude that reminiscence has caused the distress while being willing to consider such possibilities.

Reminiscence, reality orientation, cognitive training and rehabilitation, and validation therapy

Reality orientation, cognitive training and rehabilitation, and validation therapy are used only to assist people with dementia, some neurodegenerative diseases and people with acquired brain injuries (Woods *et al.* 2005). In contrast, reminiscence and life story work are used with both people who develop dementia and various other cognitive and physical conditions and people in good health. If used in dementia care then substantial adaptations are essential.

Sometimes the impression is given that reality orientation and reminiscence are synonymous. Although they share some common aspects the underlying values and theories are not identical. Cognitive training or cognitive rehabilitation is used with people who have many different kinds of neurological impairments, not only those with mild to moderate dementia. It is primarily concerned with improving specific problems concerning present cognitive functioning. These methods aim to make the most of memory and cognitive functioning by pursuing strategies that provide active training for carefully identified and focused problems by developing specific skills and providing memory aids. Validation therapy and reminiscence seek to validate a person's past but they differ in significant ways. Validation seeks to remedy or reduce distress experienced by very emotionally unstable, very old people with advanced dementia by seeking to understand whatever from their past appears to preoccupy them in the present (Clare 2005).

Reality orientation and cognitive rehabilitation

Taulbee and Folson (1966) first described reality orientation (RO) with older hospitalised psychiatric patients as a way of affirming their uniqueness and humanity, and improving their quality of life. It developed as a method for helping older people beset by failing memory to remain in touch with the present. This was attempted in two ways. The first used special classes or group activities that emphasised the here and now. The second, known as 24-hour RO, was implemented through consistent behaviour by all staff involved with the person, and the provision of reminders or memory joggers within the total care environment. These orienting reminders included notice boards, calendars, large clocks, colour coding and labelling of doors.

Earlier enthusiasm for group RO has largely disappeared because it was time consuming, relatively ineffective, disregarded the time orientation and emotional preoccupations of people with dementia and imposed the values, time perspectives and priorities of staff. It was frequently confrontational and tended to focus on lost rather than retained abilities. Its emphasis, however, on colour coding, labelling and signage has constructively influenced ideas about the design of contemporary dementia facilities.

Over recent years more sensitive techniques have evolved out of RO. The emphasis now involves a more holistic approach that is responsive to the emotional, behavioural and cognitive needs and living arrangements of individuals and their carers. These developments include cognitive stimulation, re-training and cognitive rehabilitation programmes that are designed to overcome specific memory problems of immediate concern to individuals with early-stage dementia and their carers (Clare 2005).

Cognitive rehabilitation pays attention to emotional needs, an aspect that was largely ignored in earlier RO, and also the impact of dementia on families, by developing collaborative strategies for coping with memory difficulties and other cognitive changes. Memory aids like diaries, notes and reminders, rehearsal of simple intensive training techniques and environmental modification are used to assist people with early-stage dementia to cope with specific everyday problems. They are helped to achieve clearly defined, specific outcomes that are designed to improve their current functioning and well-being. Evidence of the effectiveness of cognitive rehabilitation and training for people with early-stage Alzheimer's and vascular dementia has been assessed by Clare and Woods (2010) as insufficient in their updated Cochrane Review of efficacy. Rather than dismissing this approach altogether they suggest that further, more robust studies which remedy various identified past methodological weaknesses should be undertaken.

Validation therapy
Validation therapy is used with very old people with advanced dementia who are deeply disturbed by the resurgence of memories of loss, trauma or grief associated with events in their past lives. It can be undertaken with individuals and with groups.

The goals of validation therapy are to:

- restore a feeling of self-worth
- reduce stress
- justify living
- work towards resolving unfinished conflicts from the past
- increase verbal and non-verbal communication
- improve gait and physical well-being
- prevent withdrawal inward
- reduce the need for chemical and physical restraints. (de Klerk-Rubin 1994, 1995)

Reality concerning time and place as perceived by the person in the here and now is respected. No attempt is made to dissuade people of their erroneous views, for example that they must hurry home because their mother (long dead) is waiting for them or their own children (now independent adults) need their tea prepared. Instead the therapist listens to the words being used and the concerns being expressed. The therapist empathises with the expressed emotional needs of the person and seeks to interpret the feelings behind the words. Feil (2002) argues that this disturbed behaviour represents the struggle of the person with dementia to revert to a more secure past as a means of surviving an all too desolate threatening present. Both reminiscence and validation therapy share the assumptions that an interest in the past life of older people is important for its own sake, not just as a means of keeping them in touch with present reality, and that it is important to validate or affirm the feelings associated with the past as presented by the person with dementia. Both respect the past and use it to help the older person retain a sense of identity, personhood and security in the present. Unlike validation therapy, reminiscence is practised with people of all ages and is not restricted to very disoriented old people with advanced dementia. It has much wider objectives and uses a more varied toolkit in pursuing multiple objectives.

Conclusion

Reminiscence and related creative activities, especially music, that stimulate embodied movements such as drama, movement and mime and which stress non-verbal communication, have much to contribute to people with various kinds of dementia. Reminding carers of significant shared life experience can lessen their isolation and desperation and reassure the person with dementia that they can still communicate and share a trusting, loving relationship. In engaging in dementia-specific reminiscence work with troubled and troubling people, a detailed knowledge of each person's life history used as a tool for communicating and for understanding them in the present is invaluable. Creativity, imagination, willingness to experiment and capacity for valuing and enjoying the moment are central to working effectively with people who have dementia. Modifications of time, pace, content and duration all need careful adaptation to meet individual needs. RYCT, RO, cognitive training and rehabilitation, and validation therapy and their use with people in the early stages of dementia have been briefly summarised. Reminiscence and life story work if appropriately modified are interventions greatly valued and enjoyed by people with dementia, their families and professional carers.

Key points

- Communicating with people with dementia is possible but takes time, patience and skill.
- Non-verbal approaches are especially important in building relationships and undertaking reminiscence and life story work with individuals and small groups.
- Music is especially appreciated as a means of communication and personal enjoyment.
- Reminiscence work requires adaptation of objectives, structure, pace, duration and content for people with dementia.
- Reminiscence and linked creative activities provide constructive roles for paid and family carers and volunteers.
- Knowing a person's life story and using it as a tool for communicating helps achieve person-in-relationship-centred care.
- Reminiscence and life story work assist the retention of a sense of identity, aids communication and holds people in relationship with others.
- The key to successful work and mutual satisfaction is to appreciate and respect the individual – as he or she used to be and now is.

Application exercises

1. Select a person with dementia whose behaviour worries or intrigues you. Try by every possible means to collect detailed information about their life history. Then use your knowledge to increase the amount of time you spend together and the amount of genuine communication that takes place between you.

   Make notes about any changes you observe in your attitudes towards the person and your behaviour when you are with them.

   Discuss these changes with a fellow staff member.

2. Practise really listening (listening attentively) for five minutes to someone whom you consider is always talking in a very 'confused' way.

   Reflecting on this careful concentrated listening, what did you learn

   a. about yourself?

   b. about the person?

3. Provide an opportunity for two or three people with dementia to reminisce together for several planned sessions. Identify the rewards and the difficulties. What was achieved and for whom and at what cost?

Further reading

Bruce, E., Hodgson, S. and Schweitzer, P. (1999) *Reminiscing with People with Dementia: A Handbook for Carers.* London: Age Exchange.

Downs, M. and Bowers, B. (eds) (2008) *Excellence in Dementia Care.* Buckingham: Open University Press.

Gibson, F. and Carson, Y. (2010) 'Life story work in practice: Aiming for enduring change.' *Journal of Dementia Care 18*, 3, 20–22.

Heathcote, J. (2010) 'Life story work in practice.' *Journal of Dementia Care 18*, 1, 22–24.

Moniz-Cook, E. and Manthorpe, J. (ed.) (2009) *Early Psychosocial Interventions in Dementia.* London: Jessica Kingsley Publishers.

Schweitzer, P. and Bruce, E. (2008) *Remembering Yesterday, Caring Today.* London: Jessica Kingsley Publishers.

Chapter 12

Reminiscence with People who are Depressed

Learning outcomes

After studying this chapter you should be able to:

- recognise the significance of loss in later life
- understand about sustaining morale, different styles of reminiscing and types of reminiscers
- be able to identify whether group or individual reminiscence work is more appropriate
- appreciate the importance of using and respecting cherished objects in reminiscence
- outline the key components of a structured life review
- appreciate the importance of supervision.

Loss in later life

Depression, a disorder of mood, is the biggest threat to mental health and well-being in older people. Various biological, psychological and social factors interact to predispose, precipitate and perpetuate depression. In later life, depression may continue to affect people who have experienced earlier mental health problems. These may have been recurring depressive episodes, mood swings associated with bipolar disorder or manic depressive illness, obsessional disorders or schizophrenia. For some people depression may not occur before mid or later life as relationships and circumstances change or earlier unresolved problems re-emerge. It may be mistaken for a dementing illness, or occur simultaneously with dementia. Depression in older people too frequently goes unrecognised, unassessed and untreated.

Because much depression responds to treatment, such neglect, whether arising from ignorance or indifference, is unacceptable.

Depression is frequently, but not always, associated with the experience of loss. Loss is a universal human experience which may occur at any age. It is inevitable as people grow older. It comes in many forms and challenges people's ability to cope and to enjoy life. It may be triggered by other losses besides the death of significant people. It is not just the loss of loved ones – a partner, spouse, friends, children or grandchildren. A sense of coherence, which underlies a belief in a world that is comprehensible, manageable and meaningful, may begin to fragment under the stress of experiencing profound loss. Physical health and vigour, perhaps mental capacity as well, may decline. The roles and responsibilities once undertaken with competence and satisfaction disappear or dwindle. Many people are obliged to move house, to scale down, to shed belongings. Personally significant people, familiar places, cherished possessions, gardens, pets and pastimes that were once important and even roles and responsibilities, which although at times burdensome, nevertheless gave shape and purpose to life, may be lost.

It is impossible to understand the processes of ageing without understanding loss and bereavement. Associated feelings of anger, grief, guilt, longing, numbness, pain and shock are common and, although their intensity may lessen over time, intermittent recurrence of such deeply felt emotions, particularly if loss is cumulative as it tends to be in the lives of older people, can prove very disconcerting. (See also Chapter 15.)

Loss and relinquishment are recurring, often dominating, experiences in later life. Following the loss of a long-time spouse or partner both emotional and practical needs are considerable. While feelings of loss, grief, loneliness and depression are very common, so too are deep anxieties about coping in the immediate present while the future also seems very threatening. Throughout a long-term partnership, most couples divide up different roles and responsibilities. When one partner dies, is admitted to care or develops an incapacitating illness, the other person will be faced with taking on many new tasks and responsibilities.

But there can also be gains, development, growth, satisfaction and fresh achievements in later life, even in the face of loss. New relationships may blossom, new interests be acquired and new freedoms enjoyed. Grandchildren bring pleasure and a sense of continuity and opportunities for service to family, friends and community can provide incentives for continued social engagement.

Cognitive behavioural therapy is being increasingly used to treat depression. It concentrates on assisting people to change or modify thoughts, feelings, emotions and behaviour that are dysfunctional, meaning that these aspects are unhelpful to the person. Therapists using this approach with older people probably need to be more active throughout the counselling process than is customary with younger adults and the counselling will progress at a slower rate and pace which allows for any cognitive and sensory impairments (Gallagher-Thompson and Thompson 1996).

Cappeliez *et al.* (2008) combine cognitive behavioural therapy and reminiscence in their research-based therapeutic reminiscence work designed to assist older people who are depressed. Their re-grouping of Webster's reminiscence functions (see Chapter 4) is helpful in understanding different types of reminiscence and reminiscers' responses. They use the term cognitive reminiscence therapy which involves both cognitions and emotions and the sub-types called instrumental and integrative reminiscence.

Instrumental reminiscence encourages reminiscers to identify recollections of successful past problem solving. Integrative reminiscence encourages people to move beyond simple recall of memories and to re-appraise and integrate the memory and its associated emotions. Cappeliez *et al.*'s (2001, 2008) research uses a modified version of Birren and Cochrane's guided autobiographical writing (see Chapter 7) to conduct small groups consisting of 2–4 older people who are either in hospital or attending day centres because of depression, who meet in ten weekly 45-minute sessions. Group members prepare for each session by writing brief answers to questions about their family of origin, personal accomplishments, strengths and life experiences they wish to share with the group. Cappeliez and colleagues believe that depression results from the interplay of situational demands that an individual experiences as stressful and the negative or distorted cognitive appraisal which the person makes of the resources available to help them to cope with these stressors. The personal and environmental resources available to the individual determine how people who are depressed appraise the stressors and how they respond to them. Cappeliez and O'Rourke (2002, p.306) believe that this approach complements conventional cognitive therapy for depression and achieves 'improved self-esteem and a sense of control that reinforces a problem solving approach to life's difficulties'.

Members of Cappeliez's small groups are encouraged to engage in instrumental reminiscence. They do this by deliberately being encouraged to recall memories of past effective coping, the plans they developed to respond to these demands, the problem solving engaged in and a re-evaluation of how they either achieved their own goals, or assisted someone else to achieve goals important to that person. These recalled memories assist the depressed person to recognise and mobilise similar coping strategies and problem-solving behaviour here and now, which they are encouraged to apply to present problems. Cappeliez suggests that the vivid, concrete nature of these recalled memories of past competence is far more effective than abstract discussion of problem-solving techniques or other cognitive exercises as occurs in much contemporary counselling.

The second type of reminiscence Cappeliez and colleagues use is called integrative reminiscence which aims to re-kindle self-esteem when people are troubled by memories of past failure, wrongs inflicted, or wrongs endured. People are encouraged to recall their past and develop a fresh interpretation of it by reconsidering the possible short-term and longer-term implications of the troubling memories. Discussion within a group helps people to re-appraise their negative thoughts and feelings. By thinking, and thinking again, new insights may emerge and more generous interpretations of themselves and other people are formed. By being less hard on themselves, they may become less hard on others around them.

Even if people's present life circumstances are not particularly positive, they can be helped to leave aside past burdens imposed by memory. By combining instrumental and integrative reminiscence with supportive discussion within a small group, the recall of past coping becomes a way to re-kindle self-esteem, self-confidence and effective implementation of problem solving in the present. The past is reconfigured by being re-remembered or reconstructed and in so doing becomes a resource which enables the present to be experienced more as a challenge and less as a threat. People discover that they do not forever have to remember to keep old sores alive or to let past failures dominate their present thinking.

Coming to terms with the past improves mood and assists recovery from depression. Purposeful or intentional planned reminiscence group work or structured individual life review and life story work offers many benefits. Engaging in group reminiscence or in individual life review transforms relationships and brings people together – it reconnects them whereas depression builds walls and isolates people. Helping people to re-discover through memory work, past meaning and past sources of strength, whatever they may be – relationships, achievements, spiritual values, religion or whatever– can assist them in the present. Reminiscence and life review give people something to talk about when talking may be difficult for any number of reasons, one of which is depression with its apathy, low mood, anxiety and feelings of hopelessness. 'By talking about the past we learned to talk,' a care assistant remarked about an elderly woman who had troubled her greatly. Reminiscence is not new nor is it difficult, expensive or particularly time consuming, although training and ongoing support and supervision are necessary. It gently assists people to revisit and reconnect with their past and to see it in a new way (see Chapter 16).

Emotional support and practical coping go hand in hand if earlier but abandoned skills are to contribute to surviving loss and bereavement. Apprehension can be decreased and confidence restored if a person can be helped to recognise and rediscover through reminiscence and recall how they coped with various challenging difficulties at earlier stages of life. This can lead them to recover, revive, rehearse and re-learn earlier ways of coping. New learning can occur through the process of coping with loss and grief.

When faced with any stressful event that requires new ways of coping, reminiscence and recall are often used by people of all ages who recall past problem solving to help with present problems. Consideration of the impact of a crisis or loss and how it affects the person's own sense of self and other relationships becomes an important aspect of the mourning process. As Cappeliez and O'Rourke (2002) suggest, recalling past coping can make present problems less frightening and also provides reassurance about future coping. Reminiscence encourages people to value past competence and earlier achievements and hence value themselves, even if the present is distressing and the future threatening.

Not all reminiscence, however, is constructive. If old problems are revived without associated memories of how difficulties were overcome, a person's confidence and optimism are likely to be further undermined (Cappeliez 2009; Cappeliez, O'Rourke and

Chaudhury 2005;). For depressed people who achieve a constructive reappraisal of the past and who are able to benefit from integrative and instrumental reminiscence, a new understanding of their own self-worth and confidence will be achieved. Bohlmeijer, Smit and Cuijpers (2009) further support the value of using integrative reminiscence with community-dwelling older people with mild to moderate depression.

When faced with loss, especially loss of someone very close, people are usually bewildered. The world as they knew it has changed. They find it hard to make sense of what is happening, to feel any optimism about the future or to see the new directions that must be charted. Gradually some measure of acceptance, hope, energy and willingness to invest in new experiences gradually begins to emerge for most people. There are great individual differences in the time it takes people to adjust to loss, in how they cope and the means they use to do so. Some develop a succession of illnesses as if unexpressed painful emotions are converted into physical symptoms (Collins *et al.* 2010). Some retreat into depression while others who have an active spiritual life, a sense of coherence or a satisfying explanation about the meaning of life seem to cope much better (MacKinlay 2001). Some find unexpected comfort in being reminded of the past, as did this recently bereaved wife who had been married for over 60 years.

> I have recovered D_____ as the man I married – radical, energetic and sociable. The obituary in the newspaper described him as the man I fell in love with and married, not as he became in the last years of his life – apathetic, depressed and withdrawn. His death has given him back to me, not taken him away.

Finding meaning in life in the face of death

Various writers cited in Watt and Cappeliez (1995), and Hunt *et al.* (1997), suggest that, when advancing age brings the realisation that death is no longer far off but near at hand, people may become self-absorbed, sad or angry as old unresolved conflicts re-surface. Experiencing this urge to review one's life, although very common, is not universal. It may bring unresolved conflicts or 'unfinished business' to the surface and these sad memories may trigger serious depression or despair. Perhaps it is not so much old age as enforced retirement, at any age, or other earlier major life crisis that trigger this process of spontaneous life review. By the time people reach their seventies or eighties they possibly have less unfinished business to attend to and their life reviews have already been largely completed.

Many older people appear to be demoralised, if not clinically depressed. Cumulative loss and bereavement, or unresolved or incomplete grieving from earlier losses, may lead to a state of chronic or permanent sadness. As people age, they scarcely have time to recover from one loss before they are confronted with another. When losses come thick and fast with little recovery time in between, people may feel chronically sad, overwhelmed and unable or unwilling to invest much energy in fresh beginnings. They and their families too may need encouragement to talk together about the past and the present and to value afresh, or perhaps for the first time, achievements, joys and what life has meant at earlier stages of the life cycle and what it means now if they are gong to satisfactorily negotiate Erikson's final life stage of integrity versus despair.

Depression as a response to a diagnosis of dementia

Substantial numbers of people in the early stages of a dementing illness may be very well aware that they are losing their cognitive abilities and that their memory, independence, confidence and competence are being eroded. This can make them fearful, anxious, depressed and even terrified (Cheston and Bender 1999). The increasing emphasis on early diagnosis brings the obligation for much better provision of information, advice and support services. There need to be many more opportunities provided by well-trained workers to enable people with early and moderate dementia to review and reflect upon their life's journey which they are well able to do in order to reconsider, resolve and integrate, at least in some measure, disturbing recollections and to engage in forward planning and preparation of advanced psychological directives. (See also Chapters 11 and 15.)

Depression as a response to admission to a care home

Living in care homes and hospitals may be sufficient in itself to trigger deep regret, demoralisation or depression. The circumstances that led to the person entering care, rather than the care environment and care experience, may possibly hold the key to some residents' depression.

Regretting their inability to live independently, perhaps older people in care are more likely to complain, to make unfavourable comparisons between their present and past circumstances, and to retreat into negative repetitive reminiscence. They may use reminiscence as a way of preventing themselves from investing in the present or use it to keep alive unresolved grief or mourning unless special efforts are made to assist them to come to terms with their changed life circumstances so as to develop new sources of satisfaction despite the many changes with which they must contend (Moos and Bjorn 2006).

Housden (2009) in her review of studies concerned with reminiscence undertaken in care homes identified eight rigorous research papers dealing with the use of reminiscence in the prevention and treatment of depression in older people. She identified five key themes that either assisted or limited the effectiveness of reminiscence. These were the need to have clearly defined and accepted objectives; emphasis on the social aspects of the reminiscence occasions; opportunities for self-expression; sharing of emotions; and developing trusting relationships with group leaders.

Responses to structured life review

Individual structured life review has been shown to improve people's level of daily functioning and well-being. Haight, Michel and Hendrix (2000) followed a group of 52 mentally alert Americans who were admitted to nursing homes over a five-year period. Half were randomly assigned to undertake a structured life review (see Chapter 7) while the other half received their usual nursing care and a weekly friendly visit from a researcher. The two groups were tested on admission and then re-tested at eight weeks, one year, two years and three years. Fifty-two residents survived three years. Results showed significant persistent improvements over time for the life review group on measures of depression, life satisfaction and self-esteem.

A similar but short-term small controlled study with 30 people diagnosed with dementia who lived in four residential care homes, a dementia-specific housing with care facility and a nursing home in Northern Ireland showed significant differences between the residents who undertook a structured life review and made a simple life story book and a matched control group who received their usual care only over an eight-week period. Using a pre-test and post-test methodology, scores on measures of cognitive functioning, depression, communication and mood showed significant improvements (Haight, Gibson and Michel 2006). Haight believes life review is an effective, brief, non-threatening tool for use with a vulnerable population who are unlikely to be open to or have the opportunity to undertake psychotherapy or extensive counselling.

Intractable mental health problems

It is unlikely that life-long mental health problems will diminish with advancing age. Some depressed people who are inclined to be obsessional become preoccupied with looking back, but their guilt and bitterness remain undiminished despite repeated telling of the same story. They may become stuck over one particular episode or period and be unable to move beyond it. As Webster (1997) suggests, such people use reminiscence for 'bitterness revival', to 'keep memories of old hurts fresh'. Others may have struggled hard to reach some acceptance of their lives and they may have buried painful experiences that are now beyond conscious recall.

Some severely depressed people are so very unhappy and so absorbed in their present distress that they are unable to reminisce (James 2010). They have neither the energy nor the interest to recall the past. Their self-esteem and life satisfaction may be so precarious that they do not wish to risk re-examining in order to re-integrate a painful past. Butler (1963) suggests that older people who are unable to complete a successful life review become increasingly depressed and despairing in old age. Working with such people requires skilled professional training and is more complex than most reminiscence work.

Inexperienced reminiscence workers are often afraid they will stumble into painful aspects of a person's life and do more harm than good. It is as well for new workers to be aware of this possibility but regrettable if this anxiety prevents them from beginning to learn to practise reminiscence work. The greater risk is in doing nothing, in leaving older, isolated, miserable or demoralised people unstimulated and unsupported. Provided that a worker is empathetic, genuine and responsive and has time for listening, doing harm is unlikely. Do take notice though of what has been said already about the need for supervision and ensure that suitable support is in place.

Very occasionally, an older person may experience such painful recall and such deep distress triggered by participating in reminiscence that more skilled professional help will be required. If this happens, seek advice from senior staff, who will know how to get assistance from appropriate health and social care clinical professionals (Hawkins and Shohet 2000).

Choosing group or individual reminiscence work

Reminiscence with people who are depressed must therefore be undertaken with great care. Present depression is likely to influence the content of reminiscence. Depressed people tend to recall depressed memories, so it is important not to assume their whole life has been sad or unsatisfactory or that they have always been depressed. It may be easier for depressed people to respond to individual work where they may feel freer to talk about parts of their past that have caused them pain. In these circumstances, individual work is more likely to foster a close, confiding relationship between the older person and the reminiscence worker.

In a group, however, the depressed person, provided that they have sufficient energy to participate and do not feel out of place, may well find other members supportive and constructively reassuring. Group members may be able to challenge habitual negative interpretations and constructively suggest alternative explanations which challenge negativity and encourage the reconstruction of more positive perceptions. A group also offers the possibility of making new friends, so lessening social isolation. There can be invaluable mutual support when people discover shared experience of painful loss and transitions. Older people know more than younger people about coping with hurt, grief and loss. Pain shared in a warm accepting group may be healed or at least somewhat reduced.

In responding to depression, efforts to impart a feeling of autonomy, confidence and control are very important. Reminiscence can be used as a means of restoring some control to the person, who may at least be helped by controlling the process of recalling, reconstructing and perhaps even recording, in one way or another, their own life story.

Bohlmeijer *et al.* (2003, 2007, 2009), after reviewing a number of controlled studies, report that reminiscence and life review, especially integrative reminiscence by older people with depression, were just as effective as established drug treatments. Woods (2004), commenting on this meta analysis, cautioned that the process by which reminiscence assists in lifting depressed mood remains unclear and requires further research. If the reminiscence or life review process seems unhelpful for any individual, alternative assistance should be considered. As Coleman reminds us in Chapter 4, telling the stories of life is not always healing. For some people it may lead to further introspection or greater self-preoccupation. Professional counselling or psychotherapy of various types including approaches that rely more on non-verbal, embodied or creative forms of expression may be more effective. For some people it may be desirable to combine talking and doing therapies with medication rather than to choose one or the other. For further discussion of the use of reminiscence and related interventions for the purpose of death preparation see Chapter 15.

Using cherished objects in reminiscence

'Memorabilia' refers to things or objects that stir recollection. Sherman (1991) suggests that people who have no access to cherished objects experience a much lower mood and reduced life satisfaction compared with others in similar circumstances who can readily access objects that have special significance for them.

For everybody, depressed or not, cherished possessions – that may be of little or no monetary value – provide a sense of historical continuity, comfort, familiarity and a sense of attachment or belonging. For people who have moved from familiar to unfamiliar surroundings, perhaps by moving into a care home, such objects may be very important because they give a feeling of ownership, continuity and control, and perceived control is known to be influential in creating a sense of well-being (Perrin and May 2000).

Cherished objects also provide opportunities for both formal and informal reminiscence. They can readily engage individuals and groups in reminiscence. For example, residents in a care home could be invited to bring a special object to a group session and to talk about its associations and significance. If using personal possessions for group reminiscence be sensitive to anyone who has none available and who may be grieving for lost places and lost possessions. It is preferable if all members are able to bring an object, but if this is not possible they can be asked to describe, or perhaps draw, an object which has significance for them although it is no longer accessible. A simple effective alternative is to run a whole group session based on recalling, describing and reminiscing about objects remembered but not actually available to the group. Reminiscence work undertaken in a person's own home usually has limitless opportunities for using ready to hand memorabilia.

It is regrettable that so many people admitted to care neither bring with them nor retain cherished possessions, no matter how seemingly trivial or commonplace. Staff concerned with assessment, admission and care management need to ensure that people entering care bring cherished possessions with them. Older people, families and housing and care home managers need to understand the therapeutic importance of cherished objects and other kinds of memorabilia and they may need encouragement to ensure that both men and women entering care are not bereft of personally significant and familiar artefacts.

Conclusion

Depression in late life too often goes unrecognised and untreated. If combined with dementia, then loneliness, low mood, isolation, demoralisation, despair and troubling behaviour are almost inevitable consequences. Knowledge of each person's life history helps in understanding current behaviour and provides clues and cues for carers about how they might try to connect in the present. Individual reminiscence and structured life review and small group reminiscence are promising ways of offering assistance, challenging negative self-assessments and building new friendships. These interventions will not be suitable, appropriate or effective for everyone. They may need to be combined with medication for some people. The interventions discussed in this chapter are low risk and non-invasive. For people with depression they should only be implemented by trained, well-supported reminiscence workers. Tangible reminders in the form of cherished possessions and other memorabilia can provide a bridge between the past and the present and become a focus for present enjoyable interactions. For many people, indeed for most, the past may inevitably cast some long shadows over the present. But exploring the past also opens windows to let in fresh light that illuminates the dark places, so that the present becomes more bearable and the future looks more hopeful.

Key points

- It is important to understand about depression, grief and loss in later life.
- People need to be listened to when expressing their disappointments as well as encouraged to value their achievements.
- A combination of talking, reflection, life review and production of a tangible record can have constructive outcomes.
- People who are depressed usually recall depressed memories.
- The recall of episodes of past coping can be used as a resource for present problem solving.
- Older people and their families should be encouraged to retain cherished possessions and memorabilia because they provide continuity, familiarity, comfort and pleasure in the present.

Application exercises

1. Write down a list of key words that come to mind when you think of depression in general. Now think of a particular older person you know whom you would describe as 'depressed'. What words would you apply to them?

   Compare and contrast the two lists.

   What conclusion do you reach?

2. Considering the particular person you have thought of, can you suggest some reminiscence-type activities that might interest him or her?

   Discuss your ideas with a senior colleague, adviser, mentor or supervisor.

   If the person agrees, undertake some form of planned individual reminiscence work together.

3. What cherished memorabilia do you personally value? What steps have you taken to ensure that you will continue to have access to these cherished possessions in the future?

Further reading

Housden, S. (2009) 'The use of reminiscence in the prevention and treatment of depression in older people living in care homes.' *Groupwork 19*, 2, 28–45.

Hunt, L., Marshall, M. and Rowlings, C. (eds) (1997) *Past Trauma in Late Life*. London: Jessica Kingsley Publishers.

James, I.A. (2010) *Cognitive Behavioural Therapy with Older People*. London: Jessica Kingsley Publishers.

Kunz, J. (2007) 'Mental Health Applications of Reminiscence and Life Review.' In J. Kunz and F.G. Soltys, *Transformational Reminiscence: Life Story Work*. New York: Springer.

Manthorpe, J. and Iliffe, S. (2005) *Depression in Later Life*. London: Jessica Kingsley Publishers.

Chapter 13

Reminiscence with People with Hearing, Sight and Speech Disabilities

Learning outcomes

After studying this chapter you should be able to:

- appreciate the impact of hearing, sight and speech problems
- understand the importance of careful assessment, information and advice
- create opportunities for people with hearing, sight and speech impairments to reminisce
- be alert to the need to adapt reminiscence techniques appropriately.

The impact of sensory and speech impairment

There are people with life-long sensory and speech disabilities as well as large numbers of people who develop hearing and sight problems as they grow older. Many people who have a stroke are left with speech problems and some will also develop dementia. Frequently people will have more than one disability or impairment. People are described as deaf-blind if their combined sight and hearing impairments cause difficulties with mobility, communicating and accessing information. Multiple impairments greatly increase the likelihood of the person affected becoming socially isolated as well as having difficulty in carrying out the ordinary tasks of daily living.

Butler's book *Hearing and Sight Loss* (2004) is an excellent source of comprehensive information about sensory disabilities.

No single sensory or multiple impairment as such should automatically prevent a person from taking part in reminiscence. Provided that proper assessment and care is taken, involvement in reminiscence can lessen social isolation, restore a sense of self-worth, increase confidence and assist in improving a person's quality of life. Too frequently increasing age combined with one or more communication problems can leave people lonely and isolated, even if they are living surrounded by others, either in a family or a care facility.

Creating opportunities for participation

Careful assessment of each individual is needed if suggesting reminiscence. Consider the person's own wishes and preferences, and work out together, possibly in conjunction with relatives, or care staff, how best to enable each interested person to take part.

Many people who develop sensory disabilities in later life become acutely sensitive about their changed competence. They may also deny their difficulties, be self-conscious about using aids and they may have a higher risk of depression due to changed social factors such as increased isolation, self-imposed or otherwise, or lack of stimulation. Multiple sensory problems may be further complicated by dementia. People often complain of feeling stigmatised or ignored because other people stop trying to communicate with them. Misunderstanding or lack of effort by friends, families and professionals can thoughtlessly add to this sense of isolation and loss of confidence. Inadequate, untimely or insensitive information and absence of suitable aids and adaptations can exacerbate the difficulties.

The more limited a person's ability to communicate, the more effective individual reminiscence work, rather than group work, is likely to be. This is only a general working principle because many people with sensory impairments can and do manage to participate successfully in small groups. The presence of multiple sensory disabilities, with the possible addition of dementia, however, will add complexity to all reminiscence work with individuals, couples and small groups.

There are really three parties to any decision about whether a person with a serious sensory impairment should join a group.

1. The person concerned must be consulted. Explain carefully what is proposed. Make sure the person has understood.

2. The facilitator needs to decide whether or not he or she is sufficiently competent to cope. It may also be important to seek advice from specialist staff and if possible to seek out a co-facilitator with specialist knowledge of specific disabilities.

3. Other potential group members may need to be consulted because special demands will be made on them.

Too often, family members and professional carers make decisions on behalf of older people, especially those with sensory, speech and cognitive disabilities, and presume to speak for them, instead of enabling them to speak for themselves. Be sensitive to attitudes and actions by anyone that might restrict opportunities and exclude people from activities that they could enjoy.

The following example from a care home shows how the officer in charge thought she knew what was best for people when she advised the reminiscence worker:

> Don't bother including Mr Brown. Since his stroke he is very hard to understand and he will not be able to join in.

The worker persisted and included Mr Brown in a small group. Later he reported:

> Mr Brown was very slow to join in at first. Then I handed him the horseshoe and he became very excited and was determined to speak. He responded to everything and people were very patient listening to him.

If a potential group member is uncertain about whether or not to join a group, encourage them to come once or twice to try it out, to see how well they can manage, before making up their minds. Building self-confidence and reducing self-consciousness are very important aspects of working with people who have a disability.

Adapting reminiscence

It is especially necessary to plan carefully and to adjust the size and seating arrangements of a group, where it meets, how it is run and what multi-sensory trigger materials are used to make it possible for members with sensory problems to participate.

If a group has a mixed membership that includes some people with a disability and others without, its size and make-up need very careful thought. Small groups with co-leaders are likely to work best. Take care to ensure helpful seating arrangements and good lighting. Usually a small circle is the best arrangement. Use clear, well-modulated speech. The leader or co-leader should sit near the person with the disability and assist him or her to participate in various ways. Reminiscence groups provide many opportunities for members to help each other.

Homogeneous groups consisting of members with similar disabilities are more manageable than a heterogeneous group of people with various disabilities where it is hard to attend to everyone's different needs. If the group consists of some members with a disability and others with none, probably no more than two people with disabilities should be included.

The dual requirements to attend simultaneously to the group and to all the individuals within it are even more complex than usual if some members have a communication disability. Inexperienced leaders may find themselves initially either ignoring the needs of a single member or alternatively paying them so much attention that the needs of other group members are ignored. So much goes on, even in a very small group, that it is difficult to be aware of everything, let alone respond appropriately. Honest feedback between co-leaders as well as discussion with a supervisor or consultant is very important in developing self-awareness and a capacity to respond effectively to people who have sensory or speech disabilities or perhaps both.

Multi-sensory triggers, especially tactile triggers, are particularly helpful in stimulating discussion and assist everyone, despite their disability, to participate. If people are unable to respond to one kind of trigger, another type may prove effective, so experiment to find a person's preferred and best-functioning sensory pathway and how it may best be used to full effect.

Breaking the ice

Lack of confidence and poor motivation are the first obstacles to surmount when trying to involve people in reminiscence and low self-esteem and self-consciousness or embarrassment may hinder participation and enjoyment. People with a disability may fear making fools of themselves or being a burden to others. This means that facilitators may have to work especially hard at the beginning phase of each session to help people with hearing, speech and visual problems to feel comfortable, secure and relaxed. It may be helpful to begin each session with an exercise that relies on touch and demonstration or mime rather than on hearing, sight or speech.

Here is an example of such an exercise:

> Hide some relevant small triggers in a box or a bag (at least one for each person present) that can invite actions. The contents might be as varied as a rotary egg beater, wooden spoon, tooth or hair brush, piece of sand paper, a paint brush or a hammer. Pass the bag around so that each person in turn can select a trigger by feel and then demonstrate its use to the group, perhaps using mime rather than speech to do so.

This exercise usually captures participants' interest immediately; there is usually much laughter and guessing and soon everyone will feel confident to take their turn in having their chosen object identified. Reminiscing about the objects, their uses, their present day equivalents and associated people, places and events soon follows. Reminiscence and related activities quickly become effective ways of breaking down barriers because group reminiscence is generally so spontaneous, immediately infectious and enjoyable. The shared good fun and enthusiastic discussion encourages growth in confidence, which in turn increases participation levels.

Hearing problems

Hearing problems make participation in large groups extremely difficult. For this reason groups should be kept small. Meeting places must be free of intrusive or distracting noise and desirably fitted with a loop system to assist people who wear hearing aids. Often older people with a hearing disability feel acutely uncomfortable in surroundings where there is loud background noise. If a person has a hearing aid that magnifies background noise as well as near speech, large noisy groups are intolerable. In a small group, however, with good lighting and appropriate seating to assist lip-reading and triggers that do not rely solely on sound, many deaf people will be able to enjoy a reminiscence group. Enlarged visual and generous use of tactile triggers, which use sight, touch, taste and smell, can be very effective.

The level of frustration felt by people with acquired and progressive hearing loss is very varied. Some will enjoy being part of a small group, even if hearing is difficult. Others will be so frustrated over what they fear they are missing that their predicament is worsened. So select members very carefully and only after sensitive discussion about likely obstacles and potential benefits as well as seeking suggestions about how best to facilitate participation.

Never shout when talking to a person with a hearing impairment. Clear, careful, well-modulated speech with rephrasing is more effective. When shouting, the increased volume means that the tone is usually raised. Because many older people lose their capacity to hear high tones and consonants, shouting does not help. Rather than repetition, rephrasing which uses different sound and lip patterns will increase the likelihood of being heard and hence understood.

Lip-reading classes for older people can make good use of reminiscence. Being interested in the subject matter, participants become less self-conscious and more willing to listen attentively and speak more freely. In this way, reminiscence assists learning and lip-reading skills 'are caught, rather than taught'.

Provided that appropriate communication skills are used, people who were born deaf are as likely as anyone else to enjoy and profit from reminiscence. Ideally, trained interpreters who are also skilled reminiscence facilitators should be used, but this is not always possible. A compromise is for a reminiscence groupworker and an interpreter, sign language helper or lip speaker, as appropriate, to work together as partners. Workers must get to know each other, prepare carefully and understand and respect each other's contribution. Different skills will be needed, as hearing impaired people use many kinds of communication including lip-reading, lip-speaking, finger spelling, British Sign Language, Irish Sign Language, Sign Supported English, Paget Gorman, deaf-blind manual, block or total communication. Also remember that people from minority ethnic groups may not have mastered English or may in later life revert to their first language, and that any speech or language problems will be worsened by impaired hearing.

Amplification aids

Many different types of amplification aids are available. They include conventional and digital hearing aids, induction loops, battery-operated communicators and conversers, amplifiers and radio microphones. Advice from specialist workers such as speech and language therapists, hearing therapists, audiologists, special teachers, social workers for the deaf or medical specialists is very important before purchasing any amplification aids.

Information and specialist services and assistance vary greatly in different geographic regions although legislation, the National

Service Framework for Older People, social services guidelines for sensory impairment and the work of voluntary organisations are having an increasing impact. Advice and information is usually available from social services departments and specialist agencies such as the Royal National Institute for Deaf People (RNID), Sense, and the Disabled Living Foundation.

Visual problems

Reminiscence can be effective both with people who are born blind and those who become visually impaired in later life. Very few people who lose their sight in late life are completely blind, even when registered as severely sight impaired/blind or as sight impaired/ partially sighted. Most have some residual vision. Someone with glasses who can read only the top line of a sight chart or less at a distance of three metres could qualify for registration as sight impaired/blind by an ophthalmologist. If able to see the same line at 6 metres they may be eligible for registration as sight impaired/ partially blind. Various services and benefits are available to people so registered.

Free annual sight checks are available for anyone over 60, people over 40 with a family member with glaucoma and anyone with diabetes or who is registered as blind or partially sighted. Understanding the different effects of various common visual problems will help the reminiscence worker to understand the particular problems that people with impaired vision may be experiencing. Reminiscence workers should ask individuals in what ways they are affected and with their guidance adjust the methods and prompts used to meet particular needs and circumstances. Some common sight problems are described below in order to assist such planning.

Some common sight problems
Macular degeneration
This causes gradual loss of central vision, light sensitivity and, sometimes, distressing visual hallucinations known as Charles Bonnet syndrome. Side (peripheral) vision remains relatively normal, so that it is possible to see things out of the corner of the eye but not straight in front. 'Dry' macular degeneration is untreatable although some sudden onset 'wet' macular degeneration requires immediate specialist attention and may be treatable. Good lighting is essential; use contrasting colours, an adjustable lamp and magnifiers. Encourage viewing out of the corner of the eye rather than directly ahead.

Cataract
This means the lens of the eye becomes clouded and vision becomes blurred, misty and dim. Seeing in bright or changing light and glare becomes increasingly difficult. Onset is gradual and treatment, usually by day surgery, has a high success rate. Avoidance of glare, use of sunglasses or hat and an adjustable lamp for close work may help.

Glaucoma
This results in either the extreme edges of the field of vision fading, so vision narrows, or in blank areas developing in the centre of the field of vision. Onset is gradual and reading may still be possible although the person may bump into things or seem clumsy. They will need strong but not glaring light and colour contrast. Magnifiers may help.

Diabetic retinopathy
This can result in patchy and blurred vision that may fluctuate from day to day or even hour to hour. It may produce variable floating spots or blurring. Laser treatment may be used and sometimes regular eye drops to heal and prevent further haemorrhages on the retina are prescribed. Direct or reflected light shining straight into the eyes, or light reflected from multiple sources or broken surfaces causing glare, should be avoided; hats, sunglasses and an adjustable lamp may assist.

Retinitis pigmentosa
This is an inherited, progressive untreatable condition in which side vision or peripheral vision is lost, leaving only central vision or 'tunnel vision'. It causes night blindness, difficulty in seeing in dim or bright light and in adjusting to changes in light levels.

African-Caribbean and Asian people are more susceptible to diabetes and related visual conditions and glaucoma and may develop these conditions at a younger age. Alertness to these possibilities and particular care and attention is necessary if reminiscence work is being planned.

Using aids and adapting reminiscence
Many low vision aids, ranging from simple magnifiers to very sophisticated technological aids, are available. As with hearing

impairment, seek specialist advice. Information and assistance is available from opticians, doctors, specialist librarians, social services staff, rehabilitation officers, voluntary agencies like the Royal National Institute for the Blind (RNIB) and other specialist agencies.

For some people who become blind during their lifetime, visual images acquired from past experience and laid down in memory can be used to evoke memories. The memories of people who have acquired blindness are often crystal clear, uncluttered by more recently acquired visual images. As a consequence, these people can be invaluable historical informants.

Butler (2004) advises applying the three principles of brighter, bigger and bolder which means increased lighting, enlarged images and contrasting colours. When presenting visual triggers take account of how vision is affected by the various conditions already described and try to use people's peripheral and central vision appropriately. Objects that can be handled, tastes and smells, sounds, including reading aloud, listening to talking books and newspapers, music, audio tapes, CDs, DVDs, large print books and enlarged visual triggers can all be used effectively. Non-verbal communication will be less successful than verbal communication. Computers with the capacity to change type fonts and select contrasting colours offer versatile opportunities for accessing relevant materials. Voice-activated computer technology can also be helpful. Once again specialist workers as either advisers or reminiscence partners can be invaluable.

Speech problems

Impaired speech greatly restricts opportunities for experiencing satisfying relationships and for participating in groups. Harris (2005, p.121), a speech and language therapist, sums up the challenge: 'A speech and language disability is not one person's problem but a problem of anyone who comes into contact with that person.'

Reminiscence is a productive way of encouraging people who have impaired speech – regardless of what has caused the problem be it a stroke, Parkinson's disease, dementia, learning disability or other condition – to talk. Talking about the past is especially useful with people who require speech practice following a stroke and whose family carers find that encouraging such practice or even ordinary conversation can be a dispiriting daily struggle. Although speech can be seriously affected by a stroke, memory may or may not be affected, so either way reminiscence can be a useful tool for encouraging conversation. As with lip-reading, if people are interested in what they are talking about, the amount of conversational effort they are prepared to exert can be significantly increased. When practice brings improvement, confidence grows.

Self-consciousness, low self-esteem and lack of confidence are often forgotten in the excitement of reminiscing. The person with the speech problem is able to share their recall with others who in turn become less weary, frustrated or embarrassed by trying to persevere in conversation.

Try to obtain an assessment by a speech and language therapist through local health centres, hospitals or social services departments so that the speech difficulties of the intended participant are understood and suitable plans made. Problems with understanding (receptive) or with expressing (expressive) speech, or a mixture of both, will respond to different approaches. It is best to seek specialist advice. (Chapter 11 on dementia may also be relevant.)

Working with an individual may be more appropriate than group work, but do not automatically rule out small group reminiscence or couples' reminiscence. People should be given the chance to make their own choices, rather than have to endure decisions being imposed by a professional. For example:

> Annie, a woman of 92 living in a care home, nearly always declined to join in group activities by explaining: 'I don't speak so well since I had that stroke.' But she agreed to come to a ten- session reminiscence group to see what happened. She attended regularly showing great enjoyment but rarely spoke. In the sixth meeting she spontaneously recited a long poem about the particular part of the country where she had farmed for many years. Other group members were very moved by the poem and by Annie's perseverance in reciting it. They were quick to applaud: 'Marvellous. Marvellous' and 'She has a good memory anyhow' were two of the spontaneous compliments which Annie very much appreciated.

Some people who cannot speak coherently, perhaps because of a stroke or dementia, may still be able to sing because this area of their brain remains intact or undamaged. It is well worth experimenting with singing in case it may be possible to encourage a singing response to 'conversational' singing initiated by another person.

Conclusion

The greater the sensory and speech impairments and resulting communication problems people have, the greater the care and preparation required by the reminiscence worker who should not hesitate to seek professional advice and guidance. Careful selection and assessment will be essential. Locating and using interesting suitable multi-sensory triggers and equipment will be important. A detailed life history will help identify personal interests and relevant triggers which must then be used in ways that will enable people to respond, despite their present disabilities. Together with enthusiasm for learning about a person's past, present needs must not be neglected. Audio and visual triggers, artefacts of many different kinds, colours, shapes and textures can be used as pathways for communication depending on the nature of people's disabilities and personal preferences. Music, movement, mime, gesture, dancing, writing, drawing, photography and audio or video recordings may have a part to play. Consult the person with the impairment and, after considering the best professional advice available, the reminiscence worker should have the confidence to let his or her imagination run free. They should follow their own intuition, good sense and sensitive inclinations in developing novel approaches for people who may otherwise remain extremely isolated and intensely frustrated.

Key points

- Put the person before the disability. Listen carefully, observe closely and consult widely.
- Try not to add to the disability through ignorance, insensitivity or ineptitude.
- Do not make premature judgements that exclude people with sensory and speech impairments from opportunities to reminisce or to engage in related creative activities, particularly those that stress non-verbal forms of communication.
- Obtain specialist advice, including information about methods of communication, technical equipment, aids and adaptations.
- Seek out sensory, communication and rehabilitation specialists as co-workers.
- Develop non-verbal as well as verbal communication skills.

Application exercises

1. Identify a person with a hearing, visual or speech problem. Consider with them and other relevant people how best to provide appropriate reminiscence opportunities. Implement your ideas and then discuss the outcomes with a colleague.

2. Read about hearing, visual and speech problems at different stages of the life cycle. How can this new learning benefit the people with whom you work?

3. List ways in which you might adapt reminiscence activities to enable a person with multiple sensory disabilities to participate.

Further reading

Butler, S.J. (2004) *Hearing and Sight Loss: A Handbook for Professional Carers.* London: Age Concern Books.

Mansfield, J. (2005) *Effective Communication with People Who Have Hearing Difficulties.* Bicester: Speechmark.

Parr, S., Duchan, J. and Pound, C. (2003) *Aphasia Inside Out: Reflections on Communication Disability.* Maidenhead: Open University.

Royal College of Speech and Language Therapists (2005) *Clinical Guidelines.* Milton Keynes: Speechmark. Accessed at www.rcslt.org/members/publications/RCSLT_Clinical_Guidelines.pdf on 13/12/2010.

Chapter 14

Reminiscence with People with Learning Disabilities

Learning outcomes

After studying this chapter you should be able to:

- identify the benefits of reminiscence and life story work for people with learning disabilities
- select, adapt, preserve and use relevant triggers
- assist in making tangible records of people's life stories
- become more confident in validating disenfranchised people's experiences of bereavement, loss and grief.

The relevance of reminiscence

Reminiscence and life story work with people with learning disabilities fulfils many of the same general functions already described in earlier chapters. Each time planned reminiscence work with either individuals or groups is undertaken, the purpose and objectives need to be clear so that facilitators can explain clearly and concisely to the participants what is proposed. Published accounts of reminiscence work with people with moderate and severe learning disabilities demonstrate clearly that reminiscence work in small groups and life story work with individuals is greatly valued, indeed cherished, by many of those involved. Reminiscence enables people with learning disabilities, their families and carers to look back on their lives, recall past experience, and reflect on what the past means for themselves and for others.

Some modifications or adaptations are necessary, just as they have been necessary when working with other groups whose members have various disabilities. The guidance contained in earlier chapters on dementia, depression and sensory impairment is also relevant here. Professional staff members often report how surprised they are to find how well many people with a learning disability are able to participate in reminiscence. They stress how previously undemonstrated and unrecognised abilities emerge and personal confidence and self-esteem develop in small reminiscence groups.

Bender (1994), a clinical psychologist, identified valuable outcomes for people with moderate and severe learning disabilities who participated in reminiscence groups – which he believes should meet for at least ten sessions. He notes:

• improvement in verbal ability
• clear expression of strong emotions, particularly concerning experiences of loss
• self-control and patience, contrary to usual behaviour
• absence of socially unacceptable behaviour
• abandonment, within the group, of usual roles and habitual ways of self-presentation
• demonstration of a sense of agency, or control, over their own selves and circumstances.

The expression of loss and grief

When small reminiscence groups are held for adults with learning disabilities, many individual and collective recollections of painful memories, loss and grief are usually recounted. People with learning disabilities, including children and young people, even if living at home, are often protected from a death in the family and not given opportunities by family and professional carers to mourn with others similarly affected and to grieve openly when experiencing the death of a close relative. (See also Chapter 15 about unacknowledged or disenfranchised grief and the far-reaching implications of the death of parents for people with a learning disability.) Many also lack opportunities to talk frankly about their own experience of rejection and awareness of being 'different' and how this has affected their lives.

In the past, many people with a learning disability who are now old were admitted to large institutions, often in infancy or childhood, thereby losing contact with their families, familiar people and the neighbourhoods where they once lived. Having spent most of their lives in long-stay hospitals, they were faced in mid life or later with enormous changes as these long-stay hospitals closed. Many of these people have been relocated in the community, in care homes, hostels, small group homes or independent or semi-independent flats. For most the changes in lifestyle have been dramatic.

Opportunities to mourn both the distant past and the more recent hospital past, no matter what it was like, are essential, and yet are often denied. The long-stay mental handicap hospitals in which people spent so much of their lives need to be actively acknowledged as a significant part of life experience and hence of memory. Except for the mental handicap hospital, many people with learning disabilities have no other sense of home or special place and its associated significant people (Walmsley 2006).

Location, preservation and use of relevant triggers

So the trigger materials used to encourage reminiscence should relate to the known past, wherever it has been lived. As hospitals contract, close or are demolished and residents are transferred or resettled, it is crucial that records and personal remembered accounts of this historical heritage are preserved. Collections of photographs portraying many aspects of hospital life usually exist somewhere, because these hospitals were themselves communities. It may be possible to locate photographs of holidays, sports days, trips, fetes, farms, workshops, special occasions, staff and patients. This heritage needs to be preserved for the sake of the people whose lives it represents as well as reminders about the historical evolution of the National Health Service. For people who grew up in hospitals, staff and other patients were often a substitute family; for some, their only family. They have many stories to tell, both good and bad, happy and sad, about nurses, patients, friends, ill-treatment, kindness, punishments, jobs, recreation and the whole complex life of the hospital as a living, if frequently isolated, community.

Adapting reminiscence work

The same rules of good practice with individuals and groups apply to reminiscence work with people with learning disabilities and do not need to be repeated. Groups will require co-facilitators, and individual life story work can often be enriched and continuity assured if shared with more than one 'hearer'. When deciding on group membership, selection of people with a similar range of verbal abilities, including speed of speech, is recommended. It is not possible to be prescriptive about the number of reminiscence sessions but at least ten and often many more are suggested (Bender 2005). If it is planned to work on a group book or to assist an individual person to write their life story, several years may be necessary, as Atkinson (1994), an oral historian and reminiscence facilitator, found.

Carefully selected multi-sensory triggers are invaluable. Increased illumination and appropriate amplification are important to compensate for sight and hearing impairments. Tangible objects and associated smells are usually very evocative. Do not overload people nor bombard them with questions. Adjust the pace of working and perhaps shorten the interval between sessions. Members' recollections will spark other memories within the group so that at times a collective view, rather than a collection of individual memories, is achieved. Do not persist when attention span is limited. Be finely tuned to feelings. Help people express their pain and their frustrations and joy in their own way, at their own pace.

If people with learning disabilities are taking part in a group with other members and leaders whose life experience and abilities have been very different, be alert to any lack of common interests, shared sympathies or scapegoating that may leave an individual feeling inadequate or isolated. Alternatively, they may be surprised to discover that they too have a story to tell and others are interested in hearing it.

A group facilitated by a speech and language therapist illustrates the possibilities inherent in reminiscence work:

Reminiscence proved a most effective tool for engaging an already established mixed ability group of seven adults aged 30–65 who all lived at home and attended an adult training centre. In addition to everyone having a learning disability, one person had Down's syndrome, another was registered deaf/blind, another had cerebral palsy, several had speech impairments and another was extremely restless and difficult to engage. The speech therapist together with her assistant facilitated five weekly reminiscence sessions based on Hallowe'en, Christmas, schooldays, summer holidays and horse riding – a pastime all the group had regularly engaged in some 20 years previously when they belonged to 'Riding for the Disabled'. While all sessions were reported as successful, without doubt it was the riding session which evoked the richest memories and the most animated, instantaneous recollections. Even the names of particular favourite ponies, ridden some 20 years previously, were remembered with great pleasure. Many multi-sensory triggers were used in the session. These included photographs from earlier riding days, a saddle and bridle, grooming brushes, riding helmets and body warmers, pony nuts and, most evocative of all, the smell of hay. All members donned the riding gear, posed for their photographs and talked with rare energy and enthusiasm about their recollections.

Relatives and friends can be a crucial resource in developing life story work as Kerr (2007) and Gordon (2009) suggest but careful priming or preparation is essential if reminiscence is to be mutually beneficial. It must not be conducted as a test and even gentle quizzes can be problematic. All reminiscence activities should be failure free.

When using a family photograph album an untrained family member (or anyone else) might thoughtlessly induce disappointment by insensitive questioning. For example, 'Sure you remember that?', 'You mean you don't remember when?' 'Okay but you'll know where this is' and 'I can't believe you don't remember that holiday' will produce frustration and a profound sense of failure rather than pleasure.

Practice in using open-ended alternative questions such as 'I wonder who this might be' or 'We had a good holiday when we went to...' is strongly recommended.

Reminiscence looks back, but effective work also concerns the present and it needs to invest in the future. As people accumulate new life experiences, make a record, be building for times ahead. Take photographs, collect memorabilia, help compile a diary and preserve the life history for future use. Such work leads to person-centred care planning and relationship-centred care. When information is unearthed about earlier interests and passions it can be effectively used as a present resource to calm, comfort, distract and entertain as required. For people with a learning disability and for everyone who develops dementia, life story work needs to be adequately resourced to ensure that it is a valued core activity, not an additional expendable extra luxury.

The importance of making a tangible record

Never take for granted, or fail to appreciate, the fact that facilitators, if they choose, can write their own story. They are capable of giving their own account about how they wish to be seen and making their own record. People with learning disabilities may be able to talk about themselves but may be unable to either write or read their stories. Do not assume this means that the tangible, durable record is not valued. Its importance may be even greater than is normally thought and should never be underestimated.

The process of recall is important but so too is the sense of permanence and significance which the product or record conveys. It is immensely prized, as Doreen Cocklin testified when her revealing spoken-but-written observations were published in an anthology of prose, poetry and art by people with learning disabilities: 'This is the first time anything I have said has been written down (Atkinson and Williams 1990, p.8).' Commenting on the project in which Doreen participated, Atkinson and Williams (pp.8–9) wrote:

> The use of reminiscence enables people to emerge not as victims but as survivors; not as people deficient in skills or requisite social behaviour but as individuals with a personal history; a culture, a class, a gender, as well as impairment.

There will be a heavy reliance on the spoken, rather than the written, word. Some people may be able to write but many will need a scribe or supporter if they are to present their work in a way that makes it possible for others to appreciate it. To assist the writing, reminiscence and life story workers frequently use a tape recorder and then a 'scribe' becomes responsible for producing the record. These transcriptions need to be read back and meticulously corrected or changed to make sure the story is being told as its owner intended. A copy of the tape and the transcript should always be given to the person to keep but can then be used effectively as a prompt for further reminiscence and recall.

Community publishing and desktop publishing have meant that increasing numbers of 'silent' or 'invisible' people, not only those with learning disabilities, can now have their stories published, read and more widely appreciated. These accounts are significant contributions to developing understanding of others' experience and the ways in which marginalised, excluded and 'different' people have been denied past opportunities, so easily taken for granted by most of us.

The life story is important for the teller but it is also important for the hearer – herein lies the mutual gain for all involved, as Mabel Cooper (2005, p.36) demonstrates. She was born in 1944, admitted to a children's home as a baby, transferred, when aged 12, to St Lawrence's Mental Handicap Hospital, then, after some 20 years, relocated in the community via time spent in a half-way hostel. She then went to live with a family, chair the London Consultative Group, a self-advocacy group, visit schools to talk about her life, travel internationally and undertake consultancy and staff training. She writes:

> When I started to do my life-story, very few people like me had been able to tell their stories. I know only of one other man from the hospital who wrote about his life. I think it is important that people who lived in the institutions tell their stories because then you get to know what life was like for people like me in them days. I looked at my files at the hospital. I've got them now. Some of it is terrible – like the names what they called us in them days. But the records don't tell you what life was like on the wards. And museums don't have that information either; so if we don't tell people through our books, people won't ever know.

This work is complex and demanding. It is important to consider very carefully what people who are reminiscing actually say while they are reminiscing. Try to understand what meaning the story has for the teller in the here and now. It will be a story about the past but it will be told in a particular way in the present. This applies to all reminiscence but is particularly relevant to reminiscence with people with learning disabilities, acquired brain injury and people with dementia who are likely to have difficulty in explaining the meanings themselves.

The listener always influences the story that people tell. The teller and the hearer are co-creators of the story and no talk is meaningless. People with learning disabilities also have a story to tell. They, as much as anyone else, need someone to ask and someone to listen.

Atkinson (1998, p.73) assisted Mabel Cooper and other women with learning disabilities to write their stories and she describes the complexity of the process for both teller and hearer. Atkinson describes the process:

> Mabel Cooper, the teller: 'It was very important to me to tell them about St Lawrence's and the way it was when I was there.'

> Atkinson: '[We] have been touched, moved and angered by their revelations. These stories have helped open our eyes to what life has been like for those people who, in the earlier years of the century, had the misfortune to enter the separate and closed world of the long-stay institutions. For as we get to know those who share their reminiscences and their life stories with us, we too gain, not just knowledge or vicarious experience, but an enlargement of our capacity to feel with others whose lives have been, and may still be, very different from our own.'

Life story books

Life story work is particularly relevant because of its emphasis on making tangible, practical, written, audio or pictorial records of a person's life. These records need to be concrete, attractive, simple and direct. Creating a life story book is not a routine mechanical technique but rather a carefully focused individual intervention whose purpose is to capture the 'real' person — not to write a clinical report. Such books are relevant regardless of the level of intellectual disability of the person concerned. Hewitt (2003, p.19), a nurse educator, stresses that 'each person's life story should be approached with a fresh view to emphasise the uniqueness of that person'.

The story of a person's past life and relationships has helped to shape their present needs, desires and aspirations. If information is carefully documented in a life story book it can be a valued working tool as well as an historical record. It can:

- contribute to person-centred care planning
- help to define the person as a person, rather than as a client, patient or resident
- identify what is important to the person in the present
- serve as a communication tool for people who may find it difficult to express themselves
- help people clarify issues concerning their past and present identity that label the person as disabled
- help acknowledge past complex issues or abusive relationships
- decrease barriers and increase mutual understanding between users and service providers
- assist people to make sense of the past so as to function in the present and face the future
- identify the need for assistance to help the person deal with whatever issues emerge.

There is no one preferred format for such a book although a scrapbook approach is fairly common (see also Chapter 7). There are three stages in the process: information gathering; interpreting the information; and presenting the information.

Hewitt (2000, 2003) suggests that all information gathering interviews should be recorded and that they should be undertaken with any available person who has known the person at any stage

– family members, neighbours and staff members. The informants should be encouraged to bring any relevant photographs and artefacts to such an interview. Hewitt cautions against altering the stories in any way or being concerned about establishing accuracy. She suggests the following themes can be covered in one or two interviews with an informant whereas Atkinson stresses the importance of working directly with the subject person over a more extended period of time. They are 'evolving resources that should be added to as and when something significant happens' (Hewitt 2006, p.63). The themes are:

- birth story
- life as a baby and young child
- early memories and experiences
- favourite things
- relationships with families and friends
- places lived
- happy memories
- significant life events and other family members.

A hand-written book may be more likely to be added to in the future than either a typed or word-processed book which tends to create the impression of being finished or complete. Life story books are not the same as prescriptive care plans. It is vital that the supporter, scribe or assistant (and each word describes a different facet of the essential relationship) must create trust, respect and be clear about the task. The person being assisted must remain in control, feel secure in the process and free to withdraw at any time. The content should always be read back and adjusted according to any expressed wishes or instructions.

Futures planning

Ageing parents of people with a learning disability worry greatly about the future of their children. They are often reluctant, however, to engage in futures planning despite their preoccupation with questions about 'What will happen when I am gone?' They can be encouraged and assisted to make a record of their lives as a means of undertaking their own life review, informing future carers of their son or daughter and also providing a legacy for their adult child. They may, however, have little surplus energy to invest in the task of either futures planning or in reminiscing or life review so the reminiscence worker's first difficult task may need to focus on securing engagement or involvement. A starting point for such sensitive work could be to invite the parent to consider talking or writing about 'What I would like other people to know about our family and especially our son/daughter' (Blackman 2007). Other approaches, if they have the time and energy, could involve working with the parent to make a life story book focused on themselves or organising and annotating the family photographs, making an audio photo book or becoming involved in a guided autobiographical writing group (see Chapter 7).

Down's syndrome and dementia

Advances in medical and social care have resulted in increased life expectancy for people with learning disabilities. People with Down's syndrome are now living longer and consequently they risk developing age-related degenerative conditions, especially dementia, at an earlier age than either people with other learning disabilities or the general population (Janicki and Dalton 1999). They may also develop sight and hearing problems, thyroid malfunction or depression. Indications of dementia include the loss of various skills and alterations in mood, short-term memory and sleep patterns. People affected have many different complex and changing physical, emotional and social needs which require early diagnosis, assessment and treatment. Notwithstanding the possibility of such multiple disabilities, reminiscence and life story work can still be of immense value as a communication and relationship-building tool providing suitable adjustments are made. It is doubly important that when a learning disabled person develops dementia their carers have available detailed information about the person's past – their likes and dislikes, their behaviour and their friends and preferred activities. Otherwise present behaviour is likely to be misinterpreted.

Ideally it is desirable for people affected by dementia to receive additional support which will enable them to continue to live in their family home or a group home (Kerr 1997). Helping other residents of a group home to understand about dementia and to remember the life and times shared with the resident who develops dementia may help achieve ageing in place. Remaining in familiar surroundings with well-known companions and committed familiar staff is much preferred as inappropriate, unfamiliar or unsympathetic environments can hasten deterioration and loss of confidence. This is usually considered to be better than transfer to a care home that will accommodate substantially older people and where the special needs of a younger person with Down's syndrome or other learning disability are not always understood. Listening to and knowing each person's story helps staff carers to focus on the person rather than their disabilities (Wilkinson *et al.* 2004).

Because people with Down's suffer premature ageing and as approximately one third of them are likely to develop dementia, they, their families and professional carers should be encouraged to start a life story book as soon as possible, even in childhood, adolescence or young adulthood. It can then be added to throughout the person's lifetime as well as being used as a record, a memory jogger, a communication tool and a passport for introducing the person to hospital or care home staff should a move become necessary at any time (Hopkins 2002).

Security and continuity, based on long-established familiarity, are cornerstones of good care. If these are not possible, it is crucial for the person that new carers have a readily available tool such as a life story book from which to glean the fine-grained personal detail of a person's life – rarely found or easily located in a case record or medical notes.

Conclusion

Reminiscence and life story work, suitably modified and using various approaches and formats, are very important for people with learning disabilities of all kinds. Assisting people who have life-long intellectual disabilities to value themselves by remembering, recording and valuing their memories of past experiences is emotionally demanding work. Facilitators must respect the views and wishes of the people concerned and exercise considerable empathy, patience and personal discipline in working as supporters or enablers in the process of reminiscing and creating tangible records. It is important to begin this work as early as possible in each person's lifetime and regardless of the severity of the disability. People with Down's syndrome have an increased risk of developing early dementia and life story books can be especially useful for preserving their stories and reminding them of significant places, people, possessions and events in their lives. Such books are invaluable passports should changed circumstances make new living arrangements necessary. Family carers also may find that engaging in life review or making a life story book about themselves in addition to contributing to their child's life story book can help them to become less anxious about their own and their child's future.

Key points

- Recall of the past is important for people with learning disabilities.
- They should have their experience of grief and loss acknowledged, not denied.
- Work in imaginative creative ways to help people to achieve a tangible record.
- This record, in turn, becomes a tool for continuing communication.
- Life story work should begin early in life and be continued throughout the person's life.
- A life story book is crucial for people with Down's syndrome who have an increased risk of developing dementia at a much earlier age than the general population or people with other types of learning disability.

Application exercises

1. Identify a person with a learning disability with whom you could work to compile a record of his or her life story. Collect stories, photographs and memorabilia as well as actively preserving information now that will become part of the 'record' for the future.

2. Identify the ways you may need to adapt general and specific reminiscence work for individuals and small groups of people who have learning disabilities.

3. Reflect on the impact that the life story of a person with a learning disability has made on you.

Further reading

Atkinson, D., McCarthy, M., Walmsley, J., Cooper, M. *et al.* (eds) (2000) *Good Times, Bad Times: Women with Learning Difficulties Telling Their Stories.* Kidderminster: Bild.

Down's Syndrome Association (2004) *Ageing and Its Consequences for People with Down's Syndrome: A Guide for Parents and Carers.* London: Author.

Grey, R. (2010) *Bereavement, Loss and Learning Disability.* London: Jessica Kingsley Publishers.

Hewitt, H. (2003) 'Tell it like it is: Life story books for people with learning disabilities.' *Learning Disability Practice 6*, 8, 18–22.

Hewitt, H. (2006) *Life Story Books for People with Learning Disabilities: A Practical Guide.* Kidderminster: Bild.

Kerr, D. (2007) *Understanding Learning Disability and Dementia: Developing Effective Interventions.* London: Jessica Kingsley Publishers.

Chapter 15

Reminiscence with Terminally Ill and Bereaved People

Learning outcomes

After studying this chapter you should be able to:

- understand the relevance of reminiscence, life review and life story work to people facing terminal illness or bereavement

- appreciate the complexities of grief for bereaved people who have dementia or a learning disability

- be sensitive to the needs of children facing end of life issues themselves and also bereaved children

- realise that, although loss is an ever-present part of being human and death is one of the few certainties in life, coping with both makes heavy demands on carers, families and reminiscence workers.

Loss

Loss means to be separated from, unable to locate, or to have something taken away. Some losses are recognised and validated by society and some are not. Overcoming loss and grief is very much more complicated if the loss is denied or unregarded by others. There are many different kinds of loss besides death. These include loss of significant others, body image (how we see ourselves), relationships, money, security, pets, possessions, places, self-esteem, unfulfilled ambitions and opportunities. The actual loss itself has to be endured as well as the subsequent physical, psychological and social upsets that accompany the loss. While death is an event, bereavement is the process of experiencing the associated loss. Grief is the emotion that accompanies loss, change and readjustment and it may affect people's behaviour, physical health, mental health and sense of well-being. People experience death and bereavement and grief in many different ways and at varying speeds. Although some pattern may be recognisable (Parkes 1986) there is no such thing as a standard journey through stages of bereavement or a rigid grieve-by date. Although the intensity of the impact of the loss is likely to diminish in time, it may ebb and flow as enduring sadness, triggered by memory, can be very long lasting (see Chapter 7).

Baker (2004, p.82), who records individuals' life stories for families, writes:

> Several times an elderly person has grieved afresh at remembering the loss of a loved one very many years earlier. It had been a wound carried all that time. I remember 89 year old Ivy welled up when speaking about her father who died when she was only four years old.

Sharing memories with an empathetic listener or small group usually assists people to adjust to loss and its attendant emotions. How such opportunities are provided for children and adults facing the end of life issues will very much depend on the age and life stage that the person has reached. For some a life review, in various formats, can help to bring acceptance and readiness for death as in the process a person comes to understand what his or her life has meant or, put another way, the person comes to find meaning in life generally and, perhaps more important, meaning in their own life. Being listened to, and being able to recount aspects of the past, helps to lessen present pain and reduce current anxiety, at least to some extent, for many dying people of all ages.

Some people with a terminal diagnosis are able to live for the day and make the most of the time that is left, without experiencing overwhelming anxiety about the future. They will reach this place of acceptance – or integrity to use Erikson's term – by different routes and by diverse means. Such means can include talking with trusted people, recording a life story, undertaking a structured life review, doing guided autobiography or spiritual autobiography and engaging in painting, music or other creative activity depending upon personal values, relationships, spirituality, interests, motivation, capacity and opportunities. Acceptance of the past and understanding of its impact on the present seems to be a crucial part of grappling with the last of life's developmental challenges – achieving integrity rather than despair.

Reasons for reminiscing at times of terminal illness and bereavement

Many of the general benefits and outcomes already identified in Chapter 4 by Webster and their re-grouping by Cappeliez and colleagues into instrumental and integrative types of reminiscence are relevant. When facing death many people seek to find meaning in life and in their own life. Being listened to and being reassured by knowing that a respectful listener who may be a close friend, family member, health or social care professional or trained volunteer (as in some hospice services) is prepared to listen to whatever the dying person wishes to say about aspects of the past and possible fears about the future helps to lessen present pain and reduce current anxiety, at least to some extent. Dying people may want to express their deepest feelings, perhaps to admit past mistakes, possibly make restitution, or even forgive themselves for actual or perceived mistakes, but they may find this difficult to do. The reconstructive dynamic nature of memory can be harnessed by means of reminiscence and related creative activities to assist a terminally ill person to identify and celebrate achievements, to make the most of the time left, express regrets, make amends and say goodbye. Reminiscence helps people to recognise the values by which they have lived and the messages, stories and family history they wish to bequeath to others in tangible or intangible ways. At this time family members who encourage and share in reminiscing can show that they value the dying person and his or her lifetime journey. The benefit of doing this extends way beyond the person's death and has repercussions for the bereaved people left behind who must deal with their own feelings of grief, loss, sadness, anger and anxiety about the future and their own competence to cope.

When a couple is facing the terminal illness of one partner, joint life review work appears to be an obvious choice. This, however, may not always be the best choice. Parallel life reviews may more adequately meet the separate needs of each person. Issues of choice, autonomy and control require careful consideration. Partners may be at different stages of their shared and separate journeys into grief and may need different and separate opportunities to face its impact.

Terminally ill parents of younger children
Parents confronted with their own impending death often wish to leave behind some record or evidence of their own love and concern

for their children and their wishes for the child's future while at the same time dealing with the formidable challenges presented by their own deteriorating health. Obviously the current age of the child will influence the form and the content of such a legacy and the assistance of other adults may be required in its preparation. The following example illustrates one project designed to give such assistance but more often informal ad hoc arrangements are likely to be necessary. An example of one well-structured programme for giving such assistance is the Mothers' Living Stories Project:

> This Project aims to help mothers living with cancer or other life-threatening or chronic illness to review their lives, usually over six weekly sessions in which they are assisted by trained volunteer listeners. They are helped to audio record their living stories as legacies for their children. The process offers healing for the mother, a means of opening communication with the family and a cherished gift for children and loved ones. (Blachman 2003, p.36)

Grieving children of terminally ill or deceased parents

Children facing the inevitable death of a parent or sibling need honesty and consistency from everyone involved – near and distant relatives, family friends, professionals, and parents of childhood friends. Children's questions need sensitive but honest responses and sometimes it may not be helpful for concerned adults to wait for the child to broach the subject of a parent's illness but rather for the adult to initiate the conversation to demonstrate that they are able to appreciate the child's fears. As well as 'ordinary' conversation, storytelling, reading, drawing, painting and music and other non-verbal age-appropriate techniques are used as effective vehicles for emotional expression and communication. Participation in the funeral, use of tangible reminders of the deceased parent and encouragement to re-invest and move on in ways appropriate to the child's age, developmental stage, intellectual understanding and readiness are all important aspects of grieving and growing (Dyregov 2008). Memorabilia prepared or bequeathed by the deceased parent can become the focus for reminiscing or, if this has not been already gathered by the parent prior to his or her death, other significant adults should consider working with the bereaved child to make a memory box based on the child's shared recollections of the lost parent. Multi-sensory memorabilia will add to the usefulness of such a collection which becomes a tool for helping the child negotiate the acute stages of grief and to provide a focus for further reassurance and recollection in the years ahead.

People with dementia and terminal illness and their families

When a person has both dementia and cancer or other life threatening condition their family and professional carers face many complex demands. To provide adequate physical care, including pain relief, when communication is impaired, is demanding enough but additionally meeting the emotional needs of the person and their family members is exceedingly onerous. When people because of impaired communication, for whatever reason, are unable to verbalise their fears, hopes, discomfort and pain, depression, frustration and aggression may develop or worsen.

Many people have written about the loneliness of dying and the tendency for family members to withdraw or to distance themselves. Although improved domiciliary palliative home care is enabling more people to die at home, all too often dying remains a solitary event.

Making meaning of the sum of our days

Barrett and Soltys (2002) suggest as death nears one needs to interact to mirror back the meaning of life and so having other trusted people present is very important.

Isolation and loneliness are likely to be even greater for a person affected by dementia and their carers. Despite the aspiration and the rhetoric of person-centred care, many people with dementia are still looked upon as if they are already socially dead, emotionally disconnected, long before physical death overtakes them. While some verbal capacity remains, talking about the past may make talking in the present more possible and so help postpone the eventual parting of the ways – the end of a shared journey. When verbal capacity is lost, a person who has some knowledge of the past life of the dying person can still use that knowledge as a basis for maintaining emotional contact and possibly conversation. A family carer's own anxiety, depression, fatigue and social isolation associated with the long years of a relative's encroaching dementia are likely to be exacerbated at this time and research suggests that pre-existing depression of a carer foreshadows a poor outcome from the eventual bereavement.

A spouse facing either impending or actual bereavement of their partner is likely to gain comfort by reminiscing with their adult children or grandchildren and is a way of maintaining relationships and lessening personal grief and isolation. It can assist the grieving spouse and other friends and family members to come to terms with both the past, the present and envisioned future. They can be encouraged to recall the positives and, by honestly facing the negatives, put them to rest and remind themselves of happier times with the dying or deceased person. Engagement in a structured life review may help the bereaved person to value himself or herself at a time when self-esteem, competence and confidence are being threatened (see Chapter 7).

Spouses of people who develop dementia or other chronic terminal conditions commonly experience anticipatory grief. Long before the person dies, the carer has faced the inevitable decline when daily confronted with evidence of increasing cognitive and physical frailty. A structured life review with the carer will assist them to identify past strengths and past coping and possibly achieve resolution, and sometimes reconciliation, in the present while also accepting that the partner's eventual death is inevitable. A structured life review at this stage is an investment by the spouse in his or her own mental health if only sufficient time and energy can be found to engage in this task. Although attention to family needs is an integral part of the hospice care of cancer patients, where openness, sharing, death preparation and acknowledgement of the influence of the past on the present is encouraged in family members, similar opportunities are still too rare in dementia care services.

In the terminal stage of dementia, the person commonly will have little residual speech so two-way conversation is bound to be limited, although not always impossible. Carers have reported astonishing moments of brief psychological clarity in end-stage dementia. Usually, however, family carers will need someone else with whom to share their story at this time. This may be a professional carer, sometimes a family member or relatives of other patients or a highly skilled volunteer.

Professionals need to recognise that the family carer or significant other of a terminally ill person with dementia, who is dying from end-stage dementia or more likely from some other co-morbid condition such as pneumonia or cancer, also has complex and multiple needs. The listener must be able to encourage the family members to talk and be open to hear their stories. As well as having someone to listen to them, at this stressful time family carers need to help professional carers to understand the dying person's needs in order to ensure they are comfortable and pain free. Family members need to be kept informed of deterioration and impending death, able to ventilate their emotions and to find comfort, support and acceptance for themselves during the last days and at the time of death and in the future.

Anticipating, planning and the funeral itself, despite the associated sadness, can provide opportunities for engaging in reminiscence or life review and for celebration. Although funeral arrangements vary enormously depending on culture, religion and personal values, some family mourners find it helpful to display life story books, celebration books, photographs and memory boxes to provide a focus for reminiscence and the expression of grief, sadness and appreciation at funerals, meals or wakes (Mullan 2010).

Terminally ill children and young people and their grieving parents

Parents of dying children, it has been suggested, can be helped ahead of the child's inevitable terminal stage to endure their own grief in anticipation. As the needs of the dying child become more urgent the parent is freer and more available to the child because at least some of their grieving has now taken place. Such anticipatory grief may sometimes also apply to adult partnerships, especially where the illness is lengthy, hope of recovery long abandoned and some emotional equilibrium has replaced earlier anxiety, grief, anger and sadness. Parents who are contending with the impending or actual death of a child may fail to appreciate the needs of their other children whose own grief and loss if left unattended may re-emerge in future problem behaviour.

Music in end of life care

Music may be a source of great comfort and pleasure for dying people and their visitors. Playing music of personal relevance can open up conversation between people who may otherwise find it difficult to speak of matters of great personal importance when experiencing terminal illness. Music can provide a link between people and their families to help access memories and related emotions. It encourages conversation or provides comfort when words are unnecessary or impossible. Music can also stimulate lethargic people who may be stuck in the inertia of illness and grief. Providing music that is culturally acceptable and sensitive to the personal faith and the immediate needs of the dying person and the family can be much appreciated. Encouraging a family to compile a tape or CD of a person's preferred music, which reflects lifetime preferences at different ages and stages of life, can be a useful tool at the end of life for bringing comfort and easing grief.

Pickles (2005) suggests that we all have several 'selves' rather than just one self and that our 'musical self' remains resilient as disease, including dementia, progresses. Just as personhood depends on affirmative and responsive relationships with others who must affirm and respond, so too does the 'musical self'. To listen, sing or play alone may be helpful; shared with an understanding friend or 'musical companion' it will be much more effective and personally affirming and comforting. Music can provide an alternative means of communication when verbal communication has been lost.

Unacknowledged or disenfranchised grief

Disenfranchised grief refers to grief that is not openly acknowledged, is not socially validated or publicly acceptable and openly mourned. Just like everyone else, people with a learning disability or dementia experience loss, bereavement and grief but they are often denied the opportunity to share in and understand what has happened and to openly mourn. Similarly, divorced or separated people and gay, lesbian and bisexual partners are often excluded or not accorded a recognised place or recognition of their personal grief or loss when a past or current partner dies. Too often bereaved people have their grief denied, especially those who are overprotected by well-meaning family members. Without actively participating in mourning rituals such as sending flowers, sympathy cards, mass cards or letters or attending funerals and wakes people are left alone with their grief which can be made much more difficult to work through.

The death of a main carer can have devastating effects for people with a learning disability or dementia because in addition it may entail the loss of home, independence, familiar people, places, possessions and long-established reassuring reliable routines. Frequently it will entail relocation with all the attendant strangeness, disruption, upset and unfamiliar routines. If a main carer has a terminal illness the person with a learning disability or dementia may also be debarred from saying goodbye or preparing themselves for what is to come. Their cognitive difficulties may also limit their memory and present understanding but it is wrong to assume they have no understanding at some level, have no emotions or will soon forget the loved person. Doka (2002) suggests that people with a learning disability are disenfranchised in grief. So too are many children and many people with dementia who are likely to need special help to acknowledge and to cope openly with their grief. Sharing the experience of looking through a life story book, memory book or photographic collection in which the deceased person features, drawing, responding to poetry, music and reminiscence with an empathetic companion can all assist people to acknowledge loss and express their thoughts and feelings.

Guidance for addressing loss and grief

- respect the dying person and those who are bereaved, regardless of disability and age
- openly recognise and acknowledge grief
- provide accurate and truthful information and repeat as necessary
- adjust communication to the person's age, abilities, understanding and culture
- encourage full participation in mourning rituals
- use tangible and verbal reminders to encourage the recall of memories to assist in appreciating and celebrating the life lived
- provide continuing, respectful and appreciative support.

Conclusion

The needs of terminally ill people for reviewing their lives and preparing for death are complex and demanding. So too are the needs of family members who also may be assisted by means of reminiscence, life review and related creative activities. The terminal care of people who have both dementia and other life threatening conditions is not well understood and the needs of their family carers frequently remain inadequately addressed. Disenfranchised grief imposed on children and people with a learning disability or dementia or others whose relationships are not accepted or validated by society who are excluded from being involved in a loved person's terminal illness and associated care, death and burial and who are denied the opportunity to participate in mourning rituals, for whatever reason, are done a grave disservice. Grief denied is unlikely to be experienced constructively. Increasingly it is recognised that opportunities for engaging in conversation about the deceased person, mourning rituals and open grieving appropriate to the culture and customs of those concerned better promotes the long-term mental health of bereaved and grieving people. Without such opportunities long-enduring emotional problems and consequentially reduced well-being can result.

Key points

- It is important to create opportunities for people to tell their life stories before it is too late.
- Children of dying or deceased parents, including children who have a learning disability, require open, honest verbal and non-verbal opportunities to express their feelings in ways appropriate to their age and understanding.
- Do not attempt to prevent children or people with learning disabilities or dementia from openly participating in the funeral arrangements of a loved person.
- Disenfranchised grief can create long-enduring problems.
- Use reminiscence, life review and related creative activities to assist terminally ill people and their family carers, either separately or jointly, to value their shared lives. Wherever possible encourage the production of some form of tangible record or reminder which is age- and culturally sensitive and appropriate.

Application exercises

1. Discuss this chapter with a trusted friend or colleague. What do you think of the suggestions it contains about doing reminiscence and life review with people with a terminal illness and their family carers?

2. Identify a person who you think may be enduring disenfranchised grief. How might you seek to encourage them to share their memories of a deceased person?

3. Encourage an isolated chronically or terminally ill person to share their life story with you and if possible assist them to make a record, prepare a memory box or other such legacy for their families.

Further reading

Blackman, N. (ed.) (2007) *Loss and Learning Disability*. London: Jessica Kingsley Publishers.

Doka, K.J. (2002) *Disenfranchised Grief: New Directions, Challenges and Strategies for Practice*. Champaign, IL: Research Press.

Dyregrov, A. (2008) *Grief in Young Children: A Handbook for Adults*. London: Jessica Kingsley Publishers.

Jenkins, C. and Merry, J. (2005) *Relative Grief*. London: Jessica Kingsley Publishers.

Read, S. (1999) 'Creative Ways of Working When Exploring the Bereavement Counselling Process.' In N. Blackman (ed.) *Living with Loss: Helping People with Learning Disabilities Cope with Loss and Bereavement*. Brighton: Pavilion Publishing.

Soltys, F.G. (2007) 'Reminiscence, Grief, Loss and End of Life.' In J. Kunz and F.G. Soltys (eds) *Transformational Reminiscence: Life Story Work*. New York: Springer.

Chapter 16

Staff Development, Training, Quality, Evaluation and Research Issues

Learning outcomes

After studying this chapter you should be able to:

- develop an action plan for undertaking reminiscence work
- appreciate the importance of reminiscence training, support and supervision
- understand the importance of evaluation and research
- engage in networking and develop partnerships for sharing ideas, resources and skills
- appreciate the almost inexhaustible possibilities inherent in reminiscence work and linked creative activities.

Developing a reminiscence action plan

It is almost impossible to develop good practice and become a skilled reminiscence facilitator if you are working in isolation. Gather colleagues, mentors and friends together who will support, encourage and sustain each other's work.

Develop local resource materials. Start with work colleagues and the people who are likely to benefit from reminiscence and their families. Collect triggers that will mean something to them. Use personal triggers if possible before resorting to commercially marketed triggers. Commercial packages and Internet resources that are rapidly becoming more numerous may help in the early stages and provide ideas but some of these tend to be expensive. The same amount of money spent on acquiring local second-hand resources may give better returns.

Schools and further education colleges, community arts organisations, libraries and museums may have digital cameras, recording equipment, photographic dark rooms, colour photocopiers, computers with scanners, laser printers and other useful equipment that it may be possible to access. They will also have expertise and may be very pleased to cooperate as partners in intergenerational or community-based reminiscence projects. In return it may be possible to help identify older people willing to become historical informants, informal teachers, mentors, volunteers and research participants. It may also be possible to create opportunities for younger students to undertake community service, thereby extending their experience and helping them to fulfil various curriculum requirements or personal aspirations. Various aspects of the curriculum, not just history or community studies, can be enriched through the involvement of older people (see Chapters 8, 9 and 10).

Partnerships between different agencies that bring together the statutory and independent service sectors can release creative energy to help develop and sustain reminiscence work. Staff members from local libraries and museums can be invaluable allies. There are a lot of resources and resource people available to help develop and support good reminiscence practice but there are no short cuts to developing effective partnerships or networks.

Sharing resources

Do not hog reminiscence trigger materials or monopolise scarce resources. Try to form a local group or network which meets from time to time to share ideas, constructively criticise work in progress and exchange expertise and other assets. Reminiscence is fundamentally based on sharing personal memories and it seems natural that people who promote and practise reminiscence work should also be willing to share ideas and resources. By so doing the quality and extent of reminiscence work will grow and those involved in it will benefit personally and professionally.

This handbook has stressed cooperation. It emphasises the importance of both informal collaboration and formal supervision which itself may take different forms such as tandem or paired, team or group supervision. Reminiscence workers need to find people who can be trusted to be honest and open in offering constructive criticism because only by looking critically at actual practice will skills be developed and refined. Initial training before beginning reminiscence or life story work is important but further training needs to be linked to practice so that critical reflection becomes an integral part of ongoing development.

Inexperienced or hard-pressed reminiscence workers sometimes suggest they have run out of ideas for themes or topics and that they 'have done reminiscence'. Of course activity programmes need to be varied and refreshed rather than presented as a fixed unchangeable straitjacket. Everyone needs some variety in their life and there must always be room for imaginative creative spontaneity. The possible variations and some of the many alternatives ready to be mined are immense. The regular web-based bulletins *Elderly Care Matters* produced by Dynes and Walsh at Speechmark testify to this. For example, Issue 21, accessed on 13 December 2010 at www. speechmark.netpages/news/content.asp?PageID=86, shows how a theme can be developed for several sessions.

Developing reminiscence opportunities within people's own homes

As well as continuing to develop reminiscence work in museums, libraries, arts and community organisations, hospitals, homes, day centres and supported housing, there is an urgent need to help families, friends, volunteers and domiciliary care workers to understand how significant the past is and how they can encourage people to talk about it. As the practice of care in the community and personalised care expands and person-centred care is more widely established, more older frailer people are being assisted to remain at home and, for many, also to die at home. As a consequence, it is expected that an increasing amount of reminiscence and life story work will be undertaken with individuals and families living in the community.

Care management arrangements, personal budgets, direct payments, strict financial controls, the narrow definition of functional tasks and associated rationing of time spent by health and social care staff all exert increasing pressures. These can too often work against the development of skilled reminiscence practice. The tendency to regard care as a commodity and its recipients as consumers has many associated stultifying implications. This handbook does not apologise for arguing that older people's minds and souls (or spirits) need nourishment as much as their bodies do. Relationships nurtured by care, concern and effective communication are essential. Reminiscence and other creative activities are not expendable luxuries; they are life-sustaining essentials.

The evaluation process in reminiscence and life story work practice

If reminiscence knowledge and skills are to develop, reminiscence practitioners need to be open to having their work scrutinised by others and to be willing and able to engage in its systematic evaluation. Workers' ongoing self-evaluation throughout a project is important as has already been stressed and should involve critical examination of all the stages involved in reminiscence practice with individuals and groups. Northen and Kurland (2001, p.448) describe how in successful group work 'competence evolves out of commitment, curiosity and the thirst for knowledge'.

The following questions may help guide evaluation of a reminiscence group. The same questions could be adapted for evaluating work with an individual or couple.

1. Planning

- What needs did the participants have that led to the decision to involve them in reminiscence work?
- What did the facilitators want them to achieve?
- Were the identified objectives actually achieved?
- How well did the chosen structure match the needs and aspirations of the participants?

2. Beginning phase

- How well was an effective context for work established?
- How well did the members understand the agreed purposes and programme?
- Were ground rules established?
- How well did the ground rules contribute to or obstruct the work?

3. Middle phase

- How well did the facilitators understand each member's needs, strengths and problems?
- What was the quality of the relationship with each member and between members?
- How well did facilitators display genuineness, empathy, warmth, acceptance and respect?
- To what extent did the group achieve its intended tangible and intangible outcomes?
- To what extent did members discover common ground and respect differences?
- To what extent did facilitators feel satisfied with their exercise of reminiscence skills?

4. Ending phase

- To what extent did the facilitators adequately prepare each member and themselves for the group's ending?
- To what extent and in what ways did the group evaluate its own process and outcomes?
- What would the facilitators plan to do differently or to change in their leadership style and methods of working next time they undertake reminiscence work?

Involving group members in evaluation
It is important to involve group members in the evaluation process as this helps them to review the experience and to say what they have enjoyed, what the group has meant to them and what they would advise doing differently next time. This can be done in group discussion in the last meeting or sometimes group members are asked to complete a simple questionnaire if this is appropriate.

Reminiscence research

Every aspect of reminiscence work could benefit from further research to elucidate effective outcomes, clarify practice interventions and identify the most likely people and populations across the whole life span to gain from its use. The influence of different practice contexts, methods or approaches, modes of delivery and the relative costs and benefits incurred are other areas of inquiry. Bridging the gap between scientific labaratory-based memory studies and practice presents formidable challenges as does the huge task of translating and applying research findings to reminiscence and life story work practice in all its various aspects. The number and rigour of published studies is steadily increasing as is the range of practice applications. Important progress is being made in bridging gaps between researchers and practitioners. Slowly the value and effectiveness of reminiscence as a non-pharmacological non-invasive intervention with people who are depressed (Bohlmeijer *et al.* 2005; Cappeliez 2009; Housden 2009); people with dementia (Woods *et al.* 2005); intergenerational community work (Perlstein and Bliss 2003); arts-related reminiscence (Coaten 2009); and terminally ill people and other groups is being established by acceptably rigorous research studies. There remain many unanswered questions, however, and no doubt many questions researchers and practitioners haven't yet thought to ask. Such inquiry is the essence of developing greater understanding and more skilled practice. The growth in knowledge transfer concerning reminiscence and related creative activities is encouraging. As a low cost, low risk, widely acceptable and for the most part an overwhelmingly enjoyable experience, reminiscence and life story work are becoming established in many arts, community, educational, health and social care, museum and library contexts. Its relevance across the life span and in particular its contribution to health and well-being in later life are receiving increasing recognition although there are many problems in terms of securing adequate funding for further research and sustaining development.

Reminiscence practice with prisoners, refugees, asylum seekers, people who have endured extreme trauma and people who have AIDS-related dementia, dementia, dementia linked to learning disability, alcoholism and trauma-induced brain damage are all fruitful areas of inquiry.

Although random controlled trials and quantitative methodologies dominate research respectability, qualitative studies informed by various disciplines, for example ethnomethodology, anthropology and clinical psychology, involving individuals or small numbers of people, are yielding persuasive research results and in many reminiscence contexts are more appropriate than large quantitative studies. Much awaits further investigation, particularly concerning the role of reminiscence undertaken in different cultures and practice contexts, and with different types of reminiscers.

Different ways of training and supporting reminiscence workers and the effect of doing reminiscence work on staff, family carers and volunteers await further investigation as does the effect of reminiscence as an agent of change within whole residential care systems. Likewise the preparation and training of reminiscence workers also needs to be researched so that knowledge, understanding and skill continue to develop.

So far, most research has concentrated on outcomes with older people. The functions served by reminiscence for infants, children, adolescents and adults of all ages also require research. How memory actually works and how reminiscence processes influence the development of lifetime self-esteem and self-understanding is receiving increasing attention. The influence on memory and recall of cultural, gender, educational, age and ageing dimensions across the life cycle as well as trauma and cognitive and physical health factors continue to be fertile fields of inquiry.

The processes of reminiscence as much as its outcomes require close examination. More needs to be known about the complex interdependence of the cognitive and creative aspects of reminiscence and recall, and how to harness creativity to improve communication, nurture relationships and enhance well-being. The who, what, when, where and why of reminiscence and life review all require further systematic investigation by practitioner researchers and professional research groups which include practitioners and reminiscence participants working alongside skilled researchers.

Reminiscence training, support and supervision

The past impacts in innumerable ways on people's present lives, needs and circumstances. This means that knowledge of the past, gained by means of participation in life review, life story work and reminiscence work, can be central to understanding present functioning and meeting various aspects of present need.

Nevertheless training for reminiscence and life story work remains largely ad hoc, diffuse and educationally incoherent and mostly is limited to short courses or in-house staff development programmes. There is considerable scope for further development.

Accreditation
Skills for Care, part of the Sector Skills Council, through the Qualifications and Credit Framework (QCF), is in the process

of formulating new types of training for health and social care workers. It is responsible for determining the structure and content of vocational qualifications that meet the needs of employers, learners and users. It does not offer training courses but works closely with accrediting bodies. Open College Network, City and Guilds and several other bodies provide accreditation of courses at various levels. Reminiscence features in a number of programmes for dementia care and care of disabled people. Some of these include a reminiscence element that partially contributes to NVQ health and social care units, but NVQs are in the process of being phased out. Accredited courses are provided by various agencies including Age Exchange (www.age-exchange.org.uk), Reminiscence Network Northern Ireland (www.rnni.org) and numerous further education colleges, voluntary agencies and social enterprises throughout the UK. The University of Ulster offers a 20-credit Reminiscence module as part of its MSc in Professional Development. This module is also accredited by the Northern Ireland Social Care Council towards post-qualification registration (http://prospectus.ulster.ac.uk/course/?id=7734). A number of universities offer courses in Oral History at undergraduate and postgraduate levels. (For example see www.sussex.ac.uk/cce.)

Other courses

The Open University offers an open learning, no fee, life story work non-credit course and several other credit-bearing courses that contain relevant content. (See www.open.ac.uk.)

A large number of ad hoc training events, conferences and short courses, many of which award attendance certificates, are offered by various statutory and voluntary organisations, educational establishments and independent trainers and consultants. These training events vary greatly in level, duration, content and objectives.

Reminiscence training is often arranged in response to local requests and takes place in many different venues including health and social care agencies, libraries, museums and colleges. It may involve only staff of a specific agency or recruitment may be on a multi-agency and multi-professional basis. Local and regional training creates opportunities to establish links with other interested people who can offer mutual support and encouragement. Such networking is invaluable in developing personal confidence and competence as practitioners and for promoting the wider development of reminiscence work.

Conclusion

Reminiscence workers have to be willing to explore their own past as well as the pasts of other people if they wish to develop into competent practitioners. Close encounters of the reminiscence kind will change you – but this is a change well worth risking for your own sake and the sakes of the people with whom you work. Reminiscence is intensely practical. It alters our perspectives and enlarges our vision, interest and understanding. It extends our empathy and connects us in new ways to other people and to ourselves and our past. It helps us to care and to empower others to care.

There is much to be learned about the theory and practice of various aspects and facets of reminiscence practice and further rigorous research is greatly needed. Continued reading is essential as research findings are constantly adding to the understanding of reminiscence work and related developments. Following up the references and reading at the end of each chapter is a good way to start. When reading, try to distinguish between theory-building articles, accounts of actual reminiscence work and reports of empirical research studies. Be careful to identify what particular methods or approaches, and groups of participants, the research refers to. When applying ideas gleaned from research articles or reports of practice projects it is important to copy, as closely as possible, the same conditions described or to realise the significance of the differences or variations being introduced in order to try out the same approach. Reading about reminiscence work also provides ideas about fresh directions as well as increasing the worker's confidence and stimulating their imagination.

Remember that one meaning of 'professional' is trying to do better tomorrow what you have done today. No matter how well your work has gone so far, you will still be able, next time, to become a more attentive and empathic listener, and a more sensitive, skilled group facilitator. Consolidate your development by undertaking further reminiscence work, reading and training. In these ways you will build on what you have already learned rather than letting it become submerged or forgotten by other pressing demands on your time and attention.

Reminiscence, life story work and life review skills are comparatively easy to learn. Although reminiscence practitioners require ongoing support, supervision or mentoring, these interventions are relatively low risk, low cost and almost always enjoyable. They offer ready participation and improvements in quality of life and well-being for many different groups of people of all ages in varied circumstances while at the same time improving the communication and relationship skills, confidence and competence of formal and informal carers, professionals and volunteers.

The readers of this book who are looking to their futures as reminiscence workers with all the rich possibilities for benefiting both themselves and other people may like to complete one last exercise.

Key points

- Cooperative working, networking, supervision and sharing of resources contribute to the development of good practice.
- Training, supervision, mentoring, peer support, networking, continued reading and critical evaluation promote confidence and the acquisition of practice skills.
- Reminiscence is founded on respect for individuals, appreciation of 'difference' and recognition of our mutual interdependence as people who share a common humanity in relationship with each other.
- It demands knowledge, use of various interpersonal and organisational skills and critical reflection upon their application.
- Reminiscence, life story work and life review undertaken with individuals, families, small groups and communities requires considerable theory building and substantial further research.

Application exercise

1. Divide a sheet of paper into four columns.

(a.) In column 1 list the obstacles in your workplace or circumstances that prevent you from doing the kind of reminiscence work – whether with individuals, families, groups or communities – that you think is important to do and would like to do.

(b.) In column 2 list the personal obstacles that obstruct or inhibit you from undertaking this work.

(c.) In column 3 identify the action you intend to take to overcome the obstacles listed in columns 1 and 2.

(d.) In column 4 place a date by which you intend to have taken the actions identified in column 3

2. If possible, discuss with a colleague what you have written above.

3. In six months' time, check back. Give yourself credit and criticism for what has happened or not happened in connection with these intentions in the meantime.

Further reading

Collins, S. (2009) *Reflecting On and Developing Your Practice: A Workbook for Social Care Workers*. London: Jessica Kingsley Publishers.

Etherington, K. (2004) *Becoming a Reflexive Researcher: Using Ourselves in Research*. London: Jessica Kingsley Publishers.

Hawkins, P. and Shohet, R. (2000) *Supervision in the Helping Professions*. Maidenhead: Open University/McGraw-Hill.

Pierce, T. (2005) 'Evaluation Issues in Groupwork.' In B.K. Haight and F. Gibson (eds) *Burnside's Working with Older Adults: Group Process and Techniques*. Boston: Jones and Bartlett.

References

Age UK (2010) *The Age Agenda Bulletins.* London: Age UK.

Aldridge, D. (2000) *Music Therapy in Dementia Care.* London: Jessica Kingsley Publishers.

Aldridge, E. (2003) *How to Be a Silver Surfer: A Beginner's Guide to the Internet.* London: Age Concern.

Alzheimer's Society (2010) *Living with Dementia.* London: Alzheimer's Society. Accessed on 14/05/2010 at www.alzheimers.org.uk/mynameisnotdementia

Astell, A.J., Ellis, M.P., Bernadi, L., Alm, N. *et al.* (2010) 'Using a touch screen computer to support relationships between people with dementia and caregivers.' *Interacting with Computers 22,* 267–275.

Atkinson, D. (1994) '"I Got Put Away": Group-based Reminiscence with People with Learning Difficulties.' In J. Bornat (ed.) *Reminiscence Reviewed: Perspectives, Evaluations and Achievements.* Buckingham: Open University Press.

Atkinson, D. (1998) 'Autobiography and learning disability.' *Oral History 26,* 1, 73–80.

Atkinson, D. and Williams, F. (eds) (1990) *'Know Me as I Am': An Anthology of Prose, Poetry and Art by People with Learning Difficulties.* London: Hodder and Stoughton.

Baggot, J. (2009) *The Girl on the Wall: One Life's Rich Tapestry.* London: Icon Books.

Baker, L. (2004) 'Mixing money and memories: Running an oral history business.' *Oral History 32,* 1, 79–86.

Barrett, K.G. and Soltys, F.G. (2002) 'Geriatric social work: Supporting the patient's search for meaning.' *Geriatric Rehabilitation 17,* 4, 53–64.

Bell, V. and Troxel, D. (1997) *The Best Friends Approach to Alzheimer's Care.* Baltimore: Health Professions Press.

Bell, V. and Troxel, D. (2001) *The Best Friends Staff: Building a Culture of Care in Alzheimer's Programs.* Baltimore: Health Professions Press.

Bell, V. and Troxel, D. (2004 and 2008) *The Best Friends Book of Alzheimer's Activities.* Vols 1 and 2. Baltimore: Health Professions Press.

Bender, M. (1994) 'An Interesting Confusion: What Can We Do with Reminiscence Group Work?' In J. Bornat (ed.) *Reminiscence Reviewed: Perspectives, Evaluations and Achievements.* Buckingham: Open University Press.

Bender, M. (2005) *Therapeutic Groupwork for People with Cognitive Losses: Working with People with Dementia.* Bicester: Speechmark.

Benson, J. (2010) *Working More Creatively with Groups.* London: Routledge.

Birren, J.E. (2006) *Benefits of Memory Priming: Effects of Guided Autobiography and Reminiscence.* Mind Alert lecture in Joint Program of the American Society on Aging and MetLife Foundation. Accessed on 13/12/2010 at www.asaging.org/asav2/mindalert/pdfs/booklet_2006.pdf

Birren, J.E. and Birren, B.A. (1996) 'Autobiography: Exploring the Self and Encouraging Development.' In J. Birren, G. Kenyon, J.E. Ruth, J. Schroots and T. Svensson (eds) *Aging and Biography.* New York: Springer.

Birren, J.E. and Cochran, K. (2001) *Telling the Stories of Life through Guided Autobiography Groups.* Baltimore: Johns Hopkins University Press.

Birren, J.E. and Deutchman, D. (2005) 'Guided Autobiography Groups.' In B.K. Haight and F. Gibson (eds) *Burnside's Working with Older People: Group Process and Techniques.* Boston: Jones and Bartlett.

Blachman, L. (2003) 'Healing through Listening and Legacy.' *Conference Proceedings. International Institute of Reminiscence and Life Review.* Superior: University of Wisconsin.

Blackman, N. (2007) *Loss and Learning Disability.* London: Jessica Kingsley Publishers.

Blackwell, D. (2005) *Counselling and Psychotherapy with Refugees.* London: Jessica Kingsley Publishers.

Bluck, S. (2009) 'Living Parallel Lives: Autobiographical Memory and Reminiscence Research.' *Conference Proceedings. International Institute of Reminiscence and Life Review.* Superior: University of Wisconsin.

Bluck, S. and Alea, N. (2008) 'Remembering Being Me: The Self Continuity Function of Autobiographical Memory in Younger and Older Adults.' In F. Sani (ed.) *Self Continuity: Individual and Collective Perspectives.* New York: Psychology Press.

Bohlmeijer, E., Kramer, J. and Smit, F. Cuijpers, P. *et al.* (2009) 'The effects of integrative reminiscence on depressive symptomology and mastery of older adults.' *Journal of Community Mental Health,* Springer. Published online 24 September 2009.

Bohlmeijer, E., Roemer, M., Cuijpers, P. and Smit, F., *et al.* (2007) 'The effects of reminiscence on psychological well-being in older adults: A meta analysis.' *Aging and Mental Health* 11, 3, 291–300.

Bohlmeijer, E., Smit, F. and Cuijpers, P. (2003) 'Effects of reminiscence and life review on late-life depression: A meta analysis.' *International Journal of Geriatric Psychiatry 18,* 1088–1094.

Bornat, J. (2006) 'Reminiscence and Oral History: Parallel Universes or Shared Endeavours?' In R. Perks and A. Thomson (eds) *The Oral History Reader.* London: Routledge.

Brenner, T. and Brenner, K. (2004) 'Embracing Montessori methods in dementia care.' *Journal of Dementia Care 12,* 3, 24–27.

Bruce, E. (1998) 'Holding On to the Story: Older People, Narrative and Dementia.' In G. Roberts and J. Holmes (eds) *Healing Stories.* Oxford: Oxford University Press.

Bruce, E., Hodgson, S. and Schweitzer, P. (1999) *Reminiscing with People with Dementia: A Handbook for Carers.* London: Age Exchange.

Burns, A., Dening, T. and Lawlor, B. (2002) *Clinical Guidelines in Old Age Psychiatry.* London: Martin Donitz.

Butler, R. (1963) 'The life review: An interpretation of reminiscence in the aged.' *Psychiatry: Journal for the Study of Interpersonal Processes 6*, 1, 65–76.

Butler, R. (1995) 'The Life Review.' In B.K. Haight and J.D. Webster (eds) *The Art and Science of Reminiscing: Theory, Research, Methods and Applications.* Washington, DC: Taylor and Francis.

Butler, S.J. (2004) *Hearing and Sight Loss: A Handbook for Professional Carers.* London: Age Concern.

Cappeliez, P. (2009) 'From the Clinic to the Lab and Back: The Dialogue between Basic and Applied Research.' *Conference Proceedings. International Institute of Reminiscence and Life Review.* Superior: University of Wisconsin.

Cappeliez, P. and O'Rourke, N. (2002) 'Personality traits and existential concerns as predictors of the functions of reminiscence in older adults.' *Journal of Gerontology 57*, 116–123.

Cappeliez, P., Guindon, P. and Robitaille, A. (2008) 'Functions of reminiscence and emotional regulation among older adults.' *Journal of Aging Studies 22*, 266–272.

Cappeliez, P., Lavallee, R. and O'Rourke, N. (2001) 'Functions of reminiscence in later life as viewed by young and old adults.' *Canadian Journal on Aging 20*, 577–589.

Cappeliez, P., O'Rourke, N. and Chaudhury, H. (2005) 'The functions of reminiscence and mental health in later life.' *Aging and Mental Health 9*, 4, 295–301.

Carnwell, R. and Buchanan, J. (eds) (2004) *Effective Practice in Health and Social Care: A Partnership Approach.* Maidenhead: Open University/McGraw-Hill.

Cheston, R. and Bender, M. (1999) *Understanding Dementia: The Man with the Worried Eyes.* London: Jessica Kingsley Publishers.

Clair, A. (1996) *Therapeutic Uses of Music with Older Adults.* Baltimore: Health Professions Press.

Clare, L. (2005) 'Cognitive Rehabilitation for People with Dementia.' In M. Marshall (ed.) *Perspectives on Rehabilitation and Dementia.* London: Jessica Kingsley Publishers.

Clare, L. and Woods, R.T. (2010) 'Cognitive Rehabilitation and Cognitive Training for Early-stage Alzheimer's Disease and Vascular Dementia.' *Cochrane Database of Systemic Reviews*, Issue 4. Oxford: Cochrane Library.

Coaten, R. (2009) *Building Bridges of Understanding: The Use of Embodied Practices with Older People with Dementia and Their Care Staff as Mediated by Dance Movement Psychotherapy.* Unpublished PhD thesis. Roehampton: Roehampton University.

Coaten, R. and Warren, B. (2008) 'Dance: Developing Self-image and Self-expression through Movement.' In B. Warren (ed.) *Using the Creative Arts in Therapy and Healthcare: A Practical Introduction.* London: Routledge.

Cohen, G. (2000) *The Creative Age: Awakening Human Potential in the Second Half of Life.* New York: HarperCollins.

Cohen, G. (2004) *Uniting the Heart and Mind: Human Development in the Second Half of Life.* Mind Alert lecture in Joint Program of the American Society on Aging and MetLife Foundation. Accessed on 13/12/2010 at www.asaging.org/asav2/mindalert/pdfs/booklet_2004.pdf

Cohen, G. (2005) *The Mature Mind: The Positive Power of the Aging Mind.* New York: Basic Books.

Coleman, P.G. (1986) *Ageing and Reminiscence Processes.* Chichester: John Wiley and Sons.

Collins, D.R., Sowman, R., Tobin, F., O'Rourke, J. and Liston, R. (2010) 'YouTube: A useful tool for the older generation?' *Geriatric Medicine: Midlife and Beyond,* April, 197–199.

Cooper, M. (2005) 'Mabel Cooper – Self advocate.' *Oral History 33*, 1, 36.

Craig, C. (2005) *Meaningful Making: A Practice Guide for Occupational Therapy Staff.* Stirling: Dementia Services Development Centre.

de Klerk-Rubin, V. (1994) 'How validation is misunderstood.' *Journal of Dementia Care 2*, 2, 14–16.

de Klerk-Rubin, V. (1995) 'A safe and friendly place to share feelings.' *Journal of Dementia Care 3*, 3, 22–24.

Denis, P. and Makiwane, N. (2003) 'Stories of love, pain and courage: AIDS orphans and memory boxes.' *Oral History 31*, 2, 66–74.

Department of Health (DoH) (2009a) *Living Well with Dementia: A National Dementia Strategy.* London: Department of Health.

Department of Health (DoH) (2009b) *Living Well with Dementia: A National Dementia Strategy Implementation Plan.* London: Department of Health.

Dobrof, R. (1984) 'Introduction: A Time for Re-claiming the Past.' In M. Kaminsky (ed.) *The Uses of Reminiscence: New Ways of Working with Older Adults.* New York: Haworth.

Doel, M. (2006) *Using Groupwork.* Abingdon: Routledge.

Doka, K.J. (2002) *Disenfranchised Grief: New Directions, Challenges and Strategies for Practice.* Champaign, IL: Research Press.

Dyregov, L. (2008) *Grief in Young Children: A Handbook for Adults.* London: Jessica Kingsley Publishers.

Edwards, M. (2010) 'Derry City Council's Heritage and Museum Service.' In M. Ferguson (ed.) *A Celebration of the Valuing Heritage by Valuing Memories Project.* Belfast: Reminiscence Network Northern Ireland.

Erikson, E.H. (1982) *The Life Cycle Completed.* New York: W.W. Norton and Co.

Feil, N. (2002) *The Validation Breakthrough: Simple Techniques for Communicating with People with Alzheimer's-type Dementia.* Baltimore: Health Professions Press.

Fry, P.S. (1995) 'A Conceptual Model of Socialisation and Agenetic Trait Factors that Mediate the Development of Reminiscence Styles and Their Health Outcomes.' In B.K. Haight and J.D. Webster (eds) *The Art and Science of Reminiscing: Theory, Research Methods and Applications.* Washington, DC: Taylor and Francis.

Gallagher-Thompson, D. and Thompson, L.W. (1996) 'Applying Cognitive Behavioural Therapy to the Psychological Problems of Later Life.' In S.H. Zarit and B.G. Knight (eds) *A Guide to Psychotherapy and Aging.* Washington, DC: American Psychological Association.

Gibson, F. (2004) *The Past in the Present: Using Reminiscence in Health and Social Care.* Baltimore: Health Professions Press.

Gies, M. (2010) Interview, BBC Radio 4, 12 January.

Gilfoy, K. and Knocker, S. (2008) 'Magic across the generations.' *Journal of Dementia Care 17*, 3, 22–25.

Goldsmith, M. (1996) *Hearing the Voice of People with Dementia: Opportunities and Obstacles.* London: Jessica Kingsley Publishers.

Gordon, M. (2009) 'Using Reminiscence and Life Story Work to Support Professional and Family Carers of Adults with Both a Learning Disability and Dementia.' *Conference Proceedings. International Institute of Reminiscence and Life Review.* Superior: University of Wisconsin.

Group for Education in Museums (2010) *Best Practice Toolkit: Using Learning to Improve Health and Well-being in Older Adults.* Gillingham: GEM.

Haight, B.K. (1998) 'Use of Life Review and Life Story Books in Families with Alzheimer's Disease.' In P. Schweitzer (ed.) *Reminiscence in Dementia Care.* London: Age Exchange.

Haight, B.K. and Haight, B.S. (2007) *The Handbook of Structured Life Review.* Baltimore: Health Professions Press.

Haight, B.K., Gibson, F. and Michel, Y. (2006) 'The Northern Ireland life review/ life story book project for people with dementia.' *Alzheimer's and Dementia 2*, 56–58.

Haight, B.K., Michel, Y. and Hendrix, S. (2000) 'The extended effects of the life review in nursing home residents.' *International Journal of Aging and Human Development 50*, 2, 151–168.

Harris, J. (2005) 'Speech and Language Therapy.' In M. Marshall (ed.) *Perspectives on Rehabilitation and Dementia.* London: Jessica Kingsley Publishers.

Harris, V. (2006) *Practice and Principles in Community Development Work: Resource Pack 10.* Sheffield: Federation for Community Development Learning.

Hawkins, P. and Shohet, R. (2000) *Supervision in the Helping Professions.* Maidenhead: Open University/McGraw.

Heathcote, J. (2007) *Memories Are Made of This: Reminiscence with the Person with Dementia.* London: Alzheimer's Society.

Help the Aged (1981) *Recall.* London: Help the Aged.

Henley, A. and Schott, J. (2004) *Culture, Religion and Patient Care in a Multi-ethnic Society: A Handbook for Professionals.* London: Age Concern.

Hewitt, H. (2000) 'A life story approach for people with profound learning disabilities.' *British Journal of Nursing 9*, 2, 90–95.

Hewitt, H. (2003) 'Life story books for people with learning disability.' *Learning Disability Practice 6*, 8, 18–22.

Hewitt, H. (2006) *Life Story Books for People with Learning Disabilities: A Practical Guide.* Kidderminster: BILD.

Hopkins, G. (2002) 'This is your life.' *Community Care*, 7 March, 13, 40.

Housden, S. (2007) *Reminiscence and Lifelong Learning.* Leicester: NIACE.

Housden, S. (2009) 'The use of reminiscence in the prevention and treatment of depression in older people living in care homes.' *Groupwork 19*, 2, 28–45.

Hubbard, G., Cook, A., Tester, S. and Downs, M. (2002) 'Beyond words: Older people with dementia using and interpreting nonverbal behaviour.' *Journal of Aging Studies 16*, 155–167.

Hughes, J.C. and Baldwin, C. (2006) *Ethical Issues in Dementia Care*. London: Jessica Kingsley Publishers.

Hunt, L., Marshall, M. and Rowlings, C. (eds) (1997) *Past Trauma in Late Life*. London: Jessica Kingsley Publishers.

James, I.A. (2010) *Cognitive Behavioural Therapy with Older People*. London: Jessica Kingsley Publishers.

Janicki, M.P. and Dalton, A.J. (1999) *Dementia, Aging and Intellectual Disabilities: A Handbook*. Philadelphia: Brunner/Mazel.

Jones, G.M. and Miesen, B. (2004) *Care-giving in Dementia: Research and Applications 3*. London: Brunner-Routledge.

Keenan, B. (2009) *I'll Tell Me Ma: A Childhood Memoir*. London: Jonathan Cape.

Kemp, M. (1978) *Audio-visual Reminiscence Aids for Elderly People Including the Mentally Frail*. London: Department of Health.

Kerr, D. (1997) *Down's Syndrome and Dementia: A Practitioner's Guide*. Birmingham: Venture Press.

Kerr, D. (2007) *Understanding Learning Disability and Dementia: Developing Effective Interventions*. London: Jessica Kingsley Publishers.

Killick, J. (1994) 'There's so much more to hear when you stop to listen to individual voices.' *Journal of Dementia Care 2*, 5, 16–17.

Killick, J. (1997) *You Are Words: Dementia Poems*. London: Hawker.

Killick, J. (2005) 'Conversation.' *Journal of Dementia Care Calendar*. London: Hawker.

Killick, J. and Allan, K. (2001) *Communication and the Care of People with Dementia*. Buckingham: Open University Press.

Kitwood, T. (1997) *Dementia Reconsidered*. Buckingham: Open University Press.

Knapp, M. and Prince, M. (2007) *Dementia UK: The Full Report*. London: Alzheimer's Society.

Kurokawa, Y. (1998) 'Couple Reminiscence with Japanese Dementia Patients and Their Spouses.' In P. Schweitzer (ed.) *Reminiscence in Dementia Care*. London: Age Exchange.

Langley, D. and Langley, G. (1983) *Dramatherapy and Psychiatry*. London: Croom Helm.

Longfellow, H. www.brainyquote.com/quotes/h/henrywadsw121452.html. Accessed 30/07/2010.

Lynn, L.E. (2001) 'A Shadow Over This Day.' *Social Service Administration Magazine*. Chicago: University of Chicago Press.

MacKinlay, E. (2001) *The Spiritual Dimension of Ageing*. London: Jessica Kingsley Publishers.

Mandelstam, M. (2010) *Quick Guide to Community Care Practice and the Law*. London: Jessica Kingsley Publishers.

Marshall, M. (1998) 'How it helps to see dementia as a disability.' *Journal of Dementia Care 6*, 1, 15–17.

Marshall, W.F. (1983) *Livin' in Drumlister*. Belfast: Blackstaff Press.

McConkey, J. (1997) *The Anatomy of Memory: An Anthology*. Oxford: Oxford University Press.

McKee, K., Wilson, F., Elford, H., Goudie, F. *et al.* (2003) *Evaluating the Impact of Reminiscence on the Quality of Life of Older People.* ESRC Report. Sheffield: University of Sheffield.

Milwain, E. (2009) 'The brain and person-centred care. 1. Bringing different perspectives together.' *Journal of Dementia Care 17*, 6, 22–24.

Milwain, E. (2010a) 'The brain and person-centred care. 2. Making sense of the paradoxes of dementia.' *Journal of Dementia Care 18*, 1, 23–25.

Milwain, E. (2010b) 'The brain and person-centred care. 3. Division of function across the cerebral cortex – What it means for people with dementia.' *Journal of Dementia Care 18*, 2, 23–28.

Milwain, E. (2010c) 'The brain and person-centred care. 4. Memory, belief, emotion and behaviour.' *Journal of Dementia Care 18*, 3, 25–29.

Mistry, T. and Brown, A. (1991) 'Black/white co-working in groups.' *Groupwork 4*, 2, 101–118.

Moos, I. and Bjorn, A. (2006) 'Use of the life story in the institutional care of people with dementia: A review of intervention studies.' *Ageing and Society 26*, 431–454.

Mullan, M. (2010) 'It's a wonderful life.' *Journal of Dementia Care 18*, 3, 16–17.

Mulvenna, M. (2010) 'Better Living through Technology: The Role of Technology in Support of Reminiscence, Story Telling and Life Review.' CARDI-RNNI Your Memories Matter Conference, Belfast, 17 February 2010. Accessed on 13/12/2010 at www.cardi.ie/publications/yourmemoriesmattershowcasingreminiscenceresearchworkshoppresentations

Nolan, M.J., Brown, J., Davies, S., Nolan, J. and Keady, J. (2006) *The Senses Framework: Improving Care for Older People through a Relationship-centred Approach.* Getting Research into Practice Series. Sheffield: University of Sheffield.

Northen, H. and Kurland, R. (2001) *Social Work with Groups.* New York: Columbia University Press.

Northern Health and Social Care Trust (NHSCT) (2009) *My Life Story Book and Guidelines.* Ballymena: NHSCT.

Pallasmaa, J. (2005) *The Eyes of the Skin.* Chichester: John Wiley and Sons.

Parkes, C.M. (1986) *Bereavement: Studies of Grief in Later Life.* London: Penguin.

Payne, M. (2010) 'Enriching Now with Then: Connecting Nursing Home Residents and Staff Through Oral History.' *Research Brief.* Oxford, Ohio: Scripps Gerontology Center.

Pear, T. (1922) *Remembering and Forgetting.* London: Methuen.

Perlstein, S. and Bliss, J. (2003) *Generating Community: Intergenerational Partnerships through the Expressive Arts.* New York: Elders Share the Arts.

Perrin, T. and May, H. (2000) *Wellbeing in Dementia: An Occupational Approach for Therapists and Carers.* London: Churchill Livingstone.

Pickles, W. (2005) 'Kitwood reconsidered: Dementia, personhood and music.' *Generations Review 15*, 1, 25–27

Quas, J.A. and Fivush, R. (2009) *Emotion, Memory and Development.* New York: Oxford University Press.

Quinn, A.M. (2010) 'Living Memories Project: Warrenpoint Library.' In M. Ferguson (ed.) *A Celebration of the Valuing Heritage by Valuing Memories Project.* Belfast: Reminiscence Network Northern Ireland.

Read, P. (1996) *Returning to Nothing: The Meaning of Lost Places*. Cambridge: Cambridge University Press.

Rees, J. (2009) *Life Story Books for Adopted Children: A Family Friendly Approach*. London: Jessica Kingsley Publishers.

Rose, R. and Philpot, T. (2005) *The Child's Own Story: Life Story Work with Traumatized Children*. London: British Agencies for Adoption and Fostering (BAAF).

Rubin, D.C. (ed.) (1999) *Remembering Our Past: Studies in Autobiographical Memory*. Cambridge: Cambridge University Press.

Ryan, T. and Walker, R. (2003) *Life Story Work: A Practical Guide to Helping Children Understand Their Past*. London: British Agencies for Adoption and Fostering (BAAF).

Sampson, F. (2004) *Creative Writing in Health and Social Care*. London: Jessica Kingsley Publishers.

Savill, D. (2002) *A Time to Share: Powerful Personal Stories for Teaching History and Citizenship*. London: Age Exchange.

Schweitzer, P. (1993) *Reminiscence Projects for Children and Older People*. London: Age Exchange.

Schweitzer, P. (ed.) (1998a) *The Journey of a Lifetime*. London: European Reminiscence Network.

Schweitzer, P. (ed.) (1998b) *Reminiscence in Dementia Care*. London: Age Exchange.

Schweitzer, P. (ed.) (2004) *Mapping Memories: Reminiscence with Minority Ethnic Elders*. London: Age Exchange.

Schweitzer, P. and Bruce, E. (2008) *Remembering Yesterday, Caring Today*. London: Jessica Kingsley Publishers.

Schweitzer, P. and Trilling, A. (2005) *Making Memories Matter: The Record of a European Reminiscence Network Project*. Kassel: European Reminiscence Network.

Sherman, E. (1991) 'Reminiscentia: Cherished objects as memorabilia.' *International Journal of Aging and Human Development 38*, 89–100.

Sherman, J. (2007) *Your Digital Camera Made Easy*. London: AgeUK.

Sherman, J. (2008a) *Computing for Beginners*. London: AgeUK.

Sherman, J. (2008b) *Everyday Computing*. London: AgeUK.

Shulman, L. (2006) *The Skills of Helping Individuals, Groups, Families and Communities*. Itasca, IL: Peacock.

Stelson, C. and Dauk-Bleess, R. (2003) 'Lasting Memories: An Intergenerational Writing Project in the Elementary Classroom with Implications for Reminiscence and Life Review Work with Elders.' *Conference Proceedings. International Institute of Reminiscence and Life Review*. Superior: University of Wisconsin.

Strong, P. (2010) 'Personal Treasures Project'. M. Ferguson (ed) *A Celebration of the Valuing Heritage by Valuing Memories Projects*. Belfast Reminiscence Network Northern Ireland.

Taulbee, L.R. and Folson, J.C. (1966) 'Reality orientation for geriatric patients.' *Hospital and Community Psychiatry 17*, 133–135.

Thompson, P. (2005) *The Voice of the Past: Oral History*. Oxford: Oxford University Press.

Thomson, A. (2006) 'Anzac: Putting Popular Memory Theory into Practice in Australia.' In R. Perks and A. Thomson (eds) *The Oral History Reader*. London: Routledge.

Tuckman, B.W. and Jensen, M.A. (1984) 'Stages of small group development revisited.' *Group and Organizational Studies 2*, 419–427.

van de Kolk, B.A. (1994) 'The body keeps the score: Memory and the emerging psychology of post traumatic stress.' *Harvard Review of Psychiatry 1*, 253–265.

van Dongen, E. (2005) 'Remembering in times of misery: Can older people in South Africa "get through"?' *Ageing and Society 25*, 4, 525–541.

Walmsley, J. (2006) 'Life History Interviews with People with Learning Disabilities.' In R. Perks and A. Thomson (eds) *The Oral History Reader*. London: Routledge.

Watt, L.M. and Cappeliez, P. (1995) 'Reminiscence Interventions for the Treatment of Depression in Older Adults.' In B.K. Haight and J.D. Webster (eds) *The Art and Science of Reminiscing: Theory, Research Methods and Applications*. Washington, DC: Taylor and Francis.

Wave (2010) *Unheard Voices*. Belfast: University of Ulster (DVD).

Webster, J.D. (1997) 'The reminiscence functions scale: A replication.' *International Journal of Aging and Human Development 44*, 2, 137–149.

Wilkinson, H., Kerr, D., Cunningham, C. and Rae, C. (2004) *Home for Good? Preparing to Support People with a Learning Difficulty in Residential Settings*. Brighton: Pavilion/Joseph Rowntree.

Woods, R.T. (2004) 'Reminiscence and life review are effective therapies for depression in the elderly.' *Evidence-based Mental Health 7*, 81–83.

Woods, R.T., Spector, A.E., Jones, C.A., Orrell, M. and Davies, S.P. (2005) 'Reminiscence Therapy for Dementia.' *Cochrane Database of Systematic Reviews*, Issue 2. Chichester: John Wiley and Sons.

Yow, V. (2005) *Recording Oral History: A Guide for the Humanities and Social Sciences*. Walnut Creek, CA: Alta Mira Press.

Appendix

Recording

This section contains examples of six forms that can be used or adapted to keep a record of reminiscence work with individuals, couples and groups. Photocopying these forms is permissible but the source should be acknowledged.

Form 1: Personal history (p.290)

This summarises background information for each individual. If possible much of this information should be obtained during an initial interview if group work is intended. If working with an individual it could be used for initial selection or as an adjunct to subsequent sessions or as a guide to gathering information for a life story book.

Form 2: Individual session record (p.291)

This may be used either in individual or group sessions to summarise the response of each participant in each session. Complete after each session by rating participants' responses on a 0–4 scale.

Form 3: Reminiscence group – Group session record (p. 292)

This summarises the response of all members at each session and records attendance. Complete after each session by rating responses on a 0–4 scale.

Form 4: Reminiscence group – Facilitator's session record (p.293)

This refers to the content and process of each session. It also includes notes on debriefing and supervision connected to each session or meeting. If co-working, this form is best completed jointly by the leaders as soon as possible after each session.

Form 5: Group activity form for people with dementia (pp.294–295)

This is for use with a group of people with dementia, as an alternative to form 4.

Form 6: Consent form (p.296)

It is important to have written consent from each participant and not only if there is any likelihood that contributions may be used publicly. The consent form has two parts. Part A refers to consent to participate in reminiscence/life review/life story work and should be signed in the beginning phase, not necessarily at the first interview or group session. Part B refers to the future use of any product or outcomes. It should be anticipated with participants when a tangible product or future public use is being envisioned or planned and then completed as part of the ending phase of the work. The form can be readily adapted if necessary to suit particular individuals, groups or circumstances.

1. Personal history

Name		Date of birth		Place of birth
Source of information				
History compiled by		Date		
Preferred language			How person likes to be addressed	
First language			Country of origin	
Present marital status			Maiden name	
Date married		Place married		Spouse/ partner's name
Date bereaved				
Number of children		Number of grandchildren		Number of great grandchildren
Names/ages of children		Spouse/partner's children		Grandchildren
Spouse/partners		Spouse/partner's children		Grandchildren
Own mother's maiden name			Father's name	
Own brothers/sisters				
Spouse/partner's brothers/sisters				
Close friends and relatives				
Schools/colleges attended	Primary		Secondary	Other
Employment (i) (ii)		(iii) (iv)		
Significant places		Length of time spent there		
Reasons why significant				
Achievements or awards				
Significant events in life				
Religion	Church/mosque/temple/synagogue attended			
Personal values				
Hobbies and interests				
Favourite pets				
Musical preferences at different times throughout life				
Particular likes		Particular dislikes		
Special medical conditions (e.g. diabetes, allergies)				
Sensory impairments		Best method of communication		
Dietary restrictions/preferences				
Additional information				

Source: Michael Bender

2. Individual session record

Participant's name		Date							
Individual session	Group session	Activity							
Sessions		1	2	3	4	5	6	7	8
Willingness to join session									
0 Refused to join session									
1 Needed persuading									
2 Needed reminding									
3 Came along without prompting									
Memory									
0 No recall									
1 Recalled odd incidents									
2 Good recall without prompting									
3 Memory intact									
Interaction (spontaneity)									
0 Disruptive									
1 Offered nothing at all									
2 Spoke only if asked									
3 Responded to other participants									
4 Initiated interaction									
Participation/responsiveness (need not be verbal)									
0 No response									
1 Little response/uncooperative									
2 Active participation when prompted									
3 Active participation without prompting									
Enjoyment									
0 Showed no signs of enjoyment									
1 Occasionally showed pleasure									
2 Enjoyed majority of session									
3 Thoroughly enjoyed session									
Comments									

Source: Michael Bender

3. Reminiscence group – Group session record

	Willingness to participate	Memory	Interaction	Participation	Enjoyment
Staff					
Activity					
Date					
Members' names					
1					
2					
3					
4					
5					
6					
7					
8					
9					
10					
Main topics discussed/ material used					
Themes					
Comments					
Suggestions					

Source: Michael Bender

4. Reminiscence group – Facilitator's session record

Session no.	Date/time of session
Group facilitators	
Group members	Reasons for absences, if any
Changes since last session	
Outline of session	
Theme	Topics covered
Group activity and process	
Notes on individuals	
Interaction between group leaders	
Overall assessment of session	
Comments/suggestions	
Debriefing after session	
Supervision	

Source: Michael Bender

5. Group activity form for people with dementia

Group: _____	Session: _____	Date: _____
Leaders:		
Comments		
Group members	(Note absentees and reasons)	
A		
B		
C		
D		

1. Willingness to join group	A	B	C	D
0 Too ill (i) or absent (a)				
1 Refused to join group				
2 Needed persuading				
3 Needed reminding				
4 Came along without prompting				

2. Confused/inappropriate contributions

(Rating based on answering the question appropriately.

The number of comments is irrelevant: only rate the content.)

	A	B	C	D
0 Did not contribute anything at all or all contributions inappropriate				
1 Almost all contributions confused/inappropriate				
2 Some contributions inappropriate				
3 Most contributions appropriate				
4 All contributions appropriate				

3. Energy level	A	B	C	D
0 Doziness frequent				
1 Persistent restlessness				
2 Intermittent doziness				
3 Intermittent restlessness				
4 Appeared appropriately calm				

4. Type of reminiscence

(Positive/negative/neutral = emotion expressed by member while recalling, not content's emotion.

Member must elaborate the memory in order to be scored as 'reminiscing'.

'Yes'/'No' answers to prompts score as 'No reminiscence'.)	A	B	C	D
0 No reminiscence				
1 Recalled neutral-tone events				
2 Recalled positive-tone events				
3 Recalled negative-tone events				
4 Recalled positive and negative events				
Comments				
5. Interaction/relationships				
(Tick all appropriate boxes.)	A	B	C	D
0a Rude/inconsiderate				
0b Monopolised the session				
0c Disruptive				
0d Said nothing				
1 Spoke only to leaders or to members when prompted				
2a Made spontaneous comments to no-one in particular				
2b Made spontaneous comments to facilitator				
2c Made spontaneous comments to one other member				
3 Made spontaneous comments to other members				
4 Helped others take part				
6. Interest/participation in the group (need not be verbal)				
(Tick all appropriate boxes.)	A	B	C	D
0 Little response/uncooperative				
1 Active participation when prompted				
2 Active participation without prompting some of the time				
3 Active participation without prompting most of the time				
4 Active participation without prompting all of the time				
7. Enjoyment/satisfaction	A	B	C	D
0 Showed no signs of enjoyment/satisfaction				
1a Occasionally showed pleasure/satisfaction				
1b Showed some enjoyment/satisfaction most of the time				
2 Enjoyed/satisfied with majority of sessions				
3 Thoroughly enjoyed/satisfied with session				

Source: Thorgrimsen et al. (2002) 'The group activity form.' Journal of Occupational Therapy 65, *6, 283–287. Reprinted with permission.*

6. Consent form

A. I agree to participate in reminiscence/life review/life story work _____ (signature)		
B. Your contribution of _____ will form part of the collection of material relating to the past and present and to assist people undergoing training in reminiscence, life story work and related creative activities. This form has been drawn up in order to ensure that your contribution is only used in accordance with your wishes.		
1. May we use your contribution:		
a. for public reference?	Yes	No
b. for research purposes?	Yes	No
c. for educational use in staff development, seminars, workshops, schools, colleges, universities?	Yes	No
d. for broadcasting purposes (radio or TV)?	Yes	No
e. as a source of information that may be published?	Yes	No
f. in a public performance, display or exhibition?	Yes	No
2. May we mention your name?	Yes	No
3. Are there any further restrictions you wish to place on your material? (Please specify)		
Signature of interviewee/group member	Date	
Signature of principal family carer or partner (if appropriate)	Date	
Signature of professional carer (if appropriate)	Date	
Signature of interviewer/group facilitator	Date	
A person completing a life story book may like to say to whom they would like to leave the book.		

Source: Faith Gibson (2010) Reminiscence and Recall: A Practical Guide to Reminiscence Work. _London: Jessica Kingsley Publishers._

About the Author

Faith Gibson is an Emeritus Professor of Social Work, University of Ulster, in Northern Ireland. She trained as a social worker and teacher in the Universities of Sydney, Queensland and Chicago and is president of the Northern Ireland Reminiscence Network. Her work in social gerontology and dementia has been recognised by a Dementia Care Award from the University of Stirling, a Millennium Medal from the British Geriatrics Society and a Lifetime Achievement Award from the Northern Ireland Association of Social Workers. Her writing is based on many years of experience as a social work practitioner, teacher, reminiscence worker and researcher.

Her reminiscence publications include numerous trigger packages, training materials, articles, research reports, chapters and books, including *The Reminiscence Trainer's Pack* for Age Concern, *The Past in the Present: Using Reminiscence in Health and Social Care* for Health Professions Press, Baltimore, and, with Barbara Haight, *Burnside's Working with Older Adults: Group Process and Techniques* for Jones and Bartlett, Boston.

She writes about reminiscence, life review and life story work from wide practical experience of reminiscence work with individuals, couples and small groups, including people with dementia. She believes that skills can be learned and practice improved if reminiscence workers are willing to undertake training, read widely, apply ideas in practice, examine their work critically, and discuss it openly with peers, supervisors, mentors and other interested people.

Subject Index

Author Index